BONE IDLE

to *body idol*

Cornel Chin

Hodder Arnold

FITNESS DISCLAIMER

The information in this book is designed only to help you make informed decisions about health and fitness. It is not intended as any kind of substitute for the advice or treatment that may have been prescribed by your doctor.

Before following any of the information or recommendations in this book, you should get an assessment of your overall health from your doctor to ensure that it's safe for you to exercise.

You're solely responsible for the way you view and use the information in this book, and do so at your own risk. The author isn't responsible in any way for any kind of injuries or health problems that might occur due to using this book or following the advice in it.

Cover © Comstock Images/Getty
Jack Carey/Alamy
Illustrations by Barking Dog Art

Orders: Please contact Bookpoint Ltd, 130 Milton Park, Abingdon, Oxon OX14 4SB. Telephone: (44) 01235 827720, Fax: (44) 01235 400454. Lines are open from 9.00 to 18.00, Monday to Saturday, with a 24-hour message answering service. You can also order through our website www.hoddereducation.com

British Library Cataloguing in Publication Data
A catalogue record for this title is available from the British Library.

ISBN-10: 0 340 90799 1
ISBN-13: 9 780340 907993

First published   2006
Impression number   10 9 8 7 6 5 4 3 2 1
Year   2008   2007   2006

Typeset by Pantek Arts Ltd, Maidstone, Kent.
Printed in Great Britain for Hodder Arnold, a division of Hodder Headline,
338 Euston Road, London, NW1 3BH, by Bath Press, Bath.

Hodder Headline's policy is to use papers that are natural, renewable and recyclable products and made from wood grown in sustainable forests. The logging and manufacturing processes are expected to conform to the environmental regulations of the country of origin.

Every effort has been made to trace copyright for material used in this book. The authors and publishers would be happy to make arrangements with any holder of copyright whom it has not been possible to trace successfully by the time of going to press.

CONTENTS

CONTENTS

CONTENTS

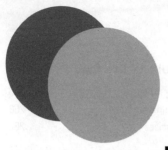

DEDICATION

This book is dedicated to my family and friends, especially to my wife Ania, whose encouragement and constant support has been invaluable. She has kept me focused. She let me be quiet when I wanted to be quiet, and when I wanted to be noisy – well, that is another story! Thank you Darling.

Thank you to my son Rafal, who constantly provides me with inspiration and motivation to always 'do better' and keeps me on my toes.

Further thanks go to Mum, Dad, my brothers Ian and Darren Chin and to my best friends Errol Arthur, David Arden and Andrew Prockter for their continued love, support and advice.

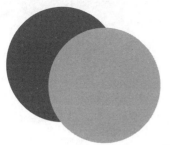

ACKNOWLEDGEMENTS

I now have the pleasant duty of thanking the several people who have contributed in one way or another to the preparation of this book. First of all, I would like to mention Liz Puttick, who not only acted as my agent, but also provided the opportunity, as well as the support and encouragement when it was most needed.

And then comes a big 'Thank you' to the great team at Hodder Education with an abundance of talent and patience. They read my drafts, understood my messages, and helped to substantially improve the presentation of the book. They are: Catherine Coe, John Hudson, Victoria Roddam, Caroline Pook and Katie Archer.

I also need to thank a wonderful man, and that was Reg Burr – he taught me many things about life. Sadly, he has passed on so my thanks go to his family, Bernice and Rosemary.

I feel compelled to mention all of my clients who offered much support and gave me 'time out' to write this book: Toni and Jerrold Assersohn, Brian Barclay, Jane Barclay, Janine Roxborough-Bunce, Rosemary Burr, Anabel Cutler, Angela Cutler, Elvie de-Rouge, David and Fozia Dick, Anthony Doran, David Gill, Henni and Irving Goldstein, Gerard Ayrton-Grime, Gilda Hamilton, Meg Jansz, Andrew Macdonald, Peter Magyar, Barbara Maher, Lynne Millar, Kate Plumb, Juliette Owide, Paula Shaw, Doris Sherwood, Siobhan Squire, Damien Tran, Labis and Sophie Tsirigotakis.

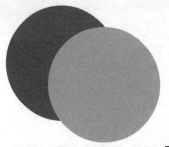

INTRODUCTION

This book is for you!

No matter what your age or level of fitness, *Bone Idle to Body Idol* is for you. It's not about a quick-fix-get-a-flat-stomach-in-one-hour-makeover, nor is it intended for you if you've already reached new heights in your pursuit of fitness. If you're physically inert and have realised that (as your biological clock is ticking away), your body will soon allow you to do even less than you can today, then this book is your life raft to a new you. It's also a book for life and is about helping you to gradually change those poor, unhealthy habits into good ones, and to help you deal with life's ups and downs.

Suit your programme to your lifestyle

Fitness is an industry that's prone to both gimmicks and quick fixes and it's no wonder that you can sometimes end up confused. High-impact aerobics? Circuit training? Low-intensity cardio? Super-slow-motion resistance training? Didn't someone say this was supposed to be fun and easy?! Well, you'll find that this book offers both ease and fun while at the same time delivering realistic and achievable results.

There are almost as many ways to exercise as there are people to do it. With some exceptions, no method is necessarily right or wrong, just different. Things to bear in mind when contemplating exercise are safety and personal risk factors, as well as individual time restraints and goals. *Bone Idle to Body Idol* will help you to devise and personalise an exercise programme that suits your lifestyle.

Moderation is everything

A well-rounded and effective exercise programme should include a moderate mix of four simple things:

- Aerobic training (aerobics means 'with air' and refers to activities such as jogging or brisk walking – see Day 56 for a detailed explanation)
- Resistance training (see Day 6 for a detailed explanation)
- Stretching (see Day 2 for a detailed explanation)
- A healthy, moderate eating plan.

It may not be over exciting and it's not headline news, but it's what works in the long term. When it comes to exercise:

'Moderation in everything' and

'If it sounds too good to be true, it probably is!'

The latest and greatest quandary among exercise gurus is aerobic exercise versus resistance training. The big question on everyone's mind seems to be, 'Which is better?' Realistically speaking, to make that choice is impossible – comparing the two is like comparing apples with oranges. Neither of them can be ruled out of a well-rounded exercise programme.

You've taken the initial steps by buying this book so you've acknowledged that you need to make some pretty serious changes in your life. You've finally discovered that the Holy Grail to getting into shape and firming up those wobbly bits isn't found in a pot of cream after all. You've realised that life isn't a rehearsal and, if left untreated, before you know it, your body will start to call it a day. This really is the only life you're going to live and it's wise to live it as long as you can, with absolute vitality.

Keep on an even keel

Perhaps you've felt that life often seems like a rollercoaster. One day you're riding high on the crest of the wave, feeling on top of the world. Then something or somebody throws a spanner in the works and sends you crashing down until you wonder if you're ever going to replenish your energy and ride the wave again. If that scenario sounds familiar, then you've got nothing to lose, but everything good and great to gain. So, read on…

You'll soon discover that this book is about setting yourself goals that are easy to achieve and are realistic, so that you won't become disheartened. It's about changing lifelong poor habits gradually, by breaking them – no matter how firmly set in concrete you think they are. It's about getting yourself active through safe, positive and beneficial exercise.

Using your *Bone Idle to Body Idol* book

The format of this book offers wise advice and serves as a 100-day diary. The first 70 days provide all the essential information you need and the next 30 days are packed with activities and tips to help you become a body idol. 100 days is long enough for you to develop many great life-changing habits and for you to get rid of the bad ones. You can even subscribe to a text messaging service to motivate and encourage you further and to ensure you achieve your goal. As you read through the material, you'll start to see a routine developing. The idea is that you don't do too much too soon or you'll get discouraged. It's best to decide for yourself what your long-term goals are, set some realistic half-way houses, and then follow your plan for that particular day. For instance, you may decide to cut out one fat or sugary food at a time and get out one floor earlier than usual when using the lift. By the end of 100 days, you'll feel a new person! You'll have formed some great new habits and changed some of the old ones. Think of this book as a stepping stone from how you are now to how you want to be. This is the start – it will work for you, so don't put it off for a moment longer!

Tips to get the best from this book

Read carefully
◆ Spend some time looking through the book to help you get a sense of what you're trying to do and why. Ensure that you take the preliminary evaluation tests before you start your exercise programme.

Focus on your goals

♦ When you start the programme, spend some time on yourself to help you focus on what you're about to embark on.

Jot things down

♦ Use the Notes pages after each chapter or buy a notebook and write down your fitness goals every day. This will act as a constant reminder and help to encourage you.

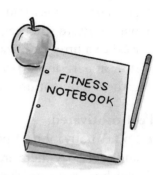

♦ Either make photocopies of the daily records from Appendix 2, or use your fitness notebook to copy out the records. Record your mood every day and how you feel after you've exercised. This will form part of your daily programme.

♦ Write down everything that you put in your mouth with complete honesty. This should include all fluids and even cigarettes. Use copies of the 'food for the day' chart from Appendix 2 for this or your fitness notebook.

♦ Note how you feel when you have the urge for unhealthy foods and how you feel if you give in to temptation or overcome it. Praise yourself if you control this urge.

♦ There are also charts in Appendix 2 for you to write down how challenging each exercise is for you, as well as your mood for the day. We're all different, so individual targets and thoughts are going to differ.

Prioritise

♦ Study the first week's programme and decide when you're going to do the exercises. You can workout at any time that suits you best. It boils down to when you feel you have both the time and the most energy. Block out time every day in your diary and do your best to prioritise the programme over everything else you're going to do. This should be an integral part of your everyday routine.

Get started now

♦ You may sometimes think that the task of transforming your fat or out-of-shape body into a toned, healthy version of its former self is insurmountable. Many people (who were probably a lot more out of shape than you at the start) have successfully dieted and exercised their way to a new look and a new way of life.

♦ Working out isn't easy or effortless, but the hardest thing to do is to get started. Once you pass that barrier, the results you feel and see will motivate you even further. Right now is where you start on the road to a fitter and healthier you! It may be a struggle at first, as the first step is always the hardest, but you'll find that the rest just gathers momentum – it will be worth it!

Feel motivated

♦ Some motivational tips are included to help you achieve your goals and every day there are some health, fitness and eating facts to keep you honed up on these subjects so you can understand and work better with your body.

Go for suppleness

♦ By the end of the first seven days, you'll be more supple and less tense. You'll also be able to walk 11 minutes a day comfortably. As you do this, you'll start feeling the positive effects of a healthier lifestyle. First, as your breathing rate increases during exercise and your heart circulates oxygen around your body, this provides a natural high. Finally, as the muscles work, they burn more calories, which results in weight loss.

Tone up

♦ By Day 10 you'll also start noticing the effects of the toning exercises (the pelvic tilts and wall press ups). These simple, yet effective exercises, which can be done anywhere and with no equipment, are designed to strengthen and tone your stomach muscles and upper body muscles.

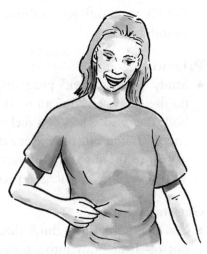

It's easy to neglect some muscle groups. These muscles play a vital part in keeping your body upright since we all do a fair amount of lifting, standing and sitting. You may not have a problem now, but as you get older, a lack of overall strength can result in lower back pain, poor posture and restricted movement in many areas.

Move forward

◆ At an early stage in your programme, you'll see that you'll be walking and toning on separate days. As you progress through your programme, new toning and strength exercises will be introduced, to help target those stubborn areas. As your strength increases, so will the number of exercises to push you comfortably and help you progress until you reach your desired shape and tone.

Daily Text Message Service

 A unique, interactive text messaging service is available★ with this book. Daily texts provide inspiration as well as key tips and advice to help you achieve your goal.

By subscribing at the beginning of a 10-day period you will receive a message each day encouraging you and supporting the guidance already given in the book for that day.

So, what are you waiting for? Text the keyword on Day 1 to 80881 to receive invaluable advice that will help you to achieve your full transformation.

★ UK only

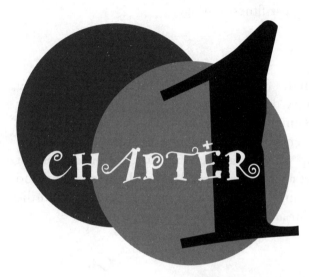

CHAPTER 1

KNOW YOURSELF:
FITNESS EVALUATION

Know yourself: fitness evaluation

Before you embark on your journey to a fitter, firmer and energetic new you, it's important to take some time to assess your current physical condition. Don't worry – it's not like a car MOT test, where you pass or fail. See it as helping to establish your overall fitness and providing a benchmark from which to start. As you become progressively healthier and more conditioned, you can monitor these changes by ongoing, regular fitness testing.

Test yourself

Firstly spend a few minutes filling in the pre-exercise questionnaire in Appendix 3. Once you've done this, you can then take the fitness test (also in Appendix 3). Remeber to tick your scores as you go along and to tot them up at the end of each test. Then see how well you did. This will not only help you to evaluate your current fitness level, but will also help you to set realistic targets and goals. These tests aren't too difficult or time-consuming. You should enjoy the challenge and the results will tell you a fair amount about the shape you're in.

Daily records

At the back of this book – in Appendix 2 – you will find some charts you can complete each day. This will help you to build a real profile of your progress.

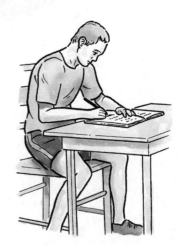

Complete the charts for today. Be honest! And don't worry – this is a base you will build and build on.

Retesting

Although you'll feel better as a result of changing your lifestyle, these changes are often hard to recognise because they occur gradually. So retest yourself after six weeks. The results will reveal how much progress you've made and will also help you to identify strengths and weaknesses so you can fine tune your exercise programme.

After your six-week retest, you may find that testing yourself every three months is more than enough. As your results and scores improve, you'll enjoy a greater sense of accomplishment and satisfaction.

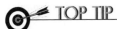 TOP TIP

- It is really helpful to spell out your main fitness goal. Make sure it is something achievable and realistic. If you can't think of one, your aim is: to jog for 30 minutes on Day 100 of this programme.

Over the rest of this week you will learn about the key elements of the *Body Idol* programme:

- Warming up
- Power walking
- Strength and toning
- Stretching.

Your notes

....

....

....

....

....

....

....

....

....

....

....

....

....

....

....

....

....

....

....

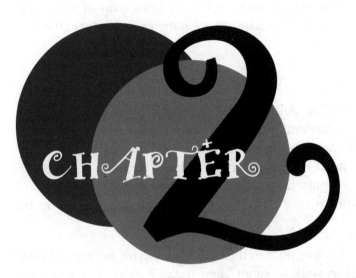

CHAPTER 2

READY, STEADY, GO!

Subscribe now to your set of 10 daily text messages. Just text 'Body Idol 1' to 80881 and receive the advice and encouragement you need to go from *Bone Idle to Body Idol*.

Each set of messages costs £1.50. Please see page xiv for full terms and conditions.

Preparing your body for exercise

Warming up should always be a part of your fitness routine. Jumping right into a workout with cold muscles can cause pain in joints and muscle. Movement literally warms up the muscles and reduces the risk of injury.

Warming up:

+ Increases circulation, delivering more oxygen to the muscles
+ Raises body temperature so the body is more efficient and less likely to suffer damage during strenuous exercise
+ Increases the heart rate in readiness for more strenuous exercise
+ Speeds up nerve impulses so that reflexes are enhanced
+ Mobilises joints so they move more freely and are less likely to be damaged.

Choose a type of warm up suited to the activity you are about to do. If you are about to walk or swim, then walk or swim to warm up – but take it slowly. Once you have activated your system, you can do a few exercises such as skipping, on-the-spot marching or step-ups to complete the process. It is then wise to add in some stretching (more on this tomorrow).

Cooling down

Cooling down after exercise is just as important as warming up.

+ Taper off your activity. For example, if you have been power walking, cool down by slowing down to a slower walk for a few minutes.
+ Finish your cool-down routine with a series of thorough and gentle stretches.

Activity

Skip for victory

Today explore the warm-up exercises explained in Appendix 1 ...

'Exercise is something good you do for yourself, that's going to last for the rest of your life.' Cornel Chin

TOP TIP 1

♦ To start limiting your alcohol consumption, figure out how many drinks you average per week, then cut that number in half.

TOP TIP 2

♦ Enjoy your exercise time as time for yourself. This is your indulgence for the day.

MYTH: You'll burn more calories jogging a mile than walking.
FACT: You burn 62 calories per 100lb body weight per mile travelled. If you weigh 150lb, you burn 93 calories per mile. The difference is, if you're jogging, you cover the distance – and burn the calories – in less time than if you're walking.

READY, STEADY, GO!

Flexibility and suppleness

When you exercise, your muscles contract and relax, contract and relax. The repeated contraction can lead to shortening of the muscles, which can lead to injury. Stretching can prevent this by:

◆ Increasing flexibility
◆ Maintaining the range of motion of muscles and joints
◆ Preparing tendons and muscles for the upcoming exercise.

To gain flexibility, you must stretch – and the proper technique is essential.

DO

◆ Use slow, static stretching techniques in which the muscle is stretched to the end of its range of motion.
◆ Ease into your stretch.
◆ Stretch to the point of slight discomfort or mild burning and then hold this position for at least 15 seconds. Hold for longer if you have time.
◆ Stretch all your major muscle groups at least once a day.

DON'T

◆ Bounce – this can cause trauma such as tearing and overstretching to the muscle fibres and tendons.
◆ Stretch forcefully.

You may be disappointed to find out how inflexible you are at first, but take heart! You should start to see improvements in your flexibility in two weeks if you stick to your daily routine.

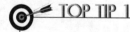

TOP TIP 1

◆ Always stay focused and tuned in to what you want to achieve!

Activity

Stretching exercises

Today you will use some stretching exercises (see Appendix 1) to get your whole body loose and limbered up.

- First warm up your body with some light exercises such as arm swings, stair step-ups or marching on the spot.

- Perform each exercise in turn, starting from your neck and gradually working down your entire body. Stand tall and concentrate on each movement as you hold, stretch and loosen your muscles. These should be executed in a slow, controlled manner. Keep your back straight, your chest high and your tummy muscles pulled in.

- As you stretch, you should feel mild discomfort. When you hold each stretch, this feeling will gradually diminish. You should find you can take the stretch a little farther, without forcing it. If you feel that the muscle being stretched begins to wobble or shake, ease off a little until the feeling has gone.

TOP TIP 2

- Try consuming one less cup of coffee or tea today.

MYTH: You burn more fat if you exercise on an empty stomach.
FACT: Exercising on an empty stomach does not affect how you lose weight – and you need energy to exercise. You should at least drink a glass of juice before an early morning workout.

READY, STEADY, GO!

9

Walk the walk!

If there's one thing our bodies were meant to do, it's to walk.

Studies show that when done briskly on a regular schedule, walking can improve the body's ability to consume oxygen during exertion, lower the resting heart rate, reduce blood pressure and increase the efficiency of the heart and lungs. It also improves muscle tone and strength and relieves stress. What's more, there is little risk of injury from walking and it can be done practically anywhere.

Here are some tips to help you develop an easy walking style:

♦ Take long, easy strides, but don't strain for distance. When walking on hills or at a very rapid pace, lean forward slightly and 'pump' with your arms.
♦ Breathe deeply and regularly.
♦ You should just be able to carry on a conversation while walking. If you're too breathless to talk, you're going too fast. If you're talking too easily, step up your pace.
♦ As you become fitter, increase the challenge by walking on hills, swinging your arms, holding weights or increasing your speed.

Gear up

Be sure to select comfortable footwear. A walking shoe should have arch supports and elevate the heel 1/2 to 3/4 of an inch above the sole of the foot. Choose a shoe with uppers made of materials that 'breathe', such as leather or nylon mesh.

Another item to consider is a pedometer. Models that just track your steps are small, easy to use, very inexpensive, and can serve as an effective motivational gadget.

'A vigorous five-mile walk will do more good for an unhappy but otherwise healthy adult than all the medicine and psychology in the world.' Paul Dudley White, American Cardiologist

Activity

Cardio 8-minute walk

Put on your watch and time yourself. Today you embark on your journey to fitness and well-being. Enjoy the sensation of being outside and the general feeling of moving your body as you walk. Breathe in deeply and exhale slowly – take in the fresh air!

After you've completed your walk, spend some time stretching out your leg muscles. Feel the tension and stresses of the previous days easing with each second that passes.

TOP TIP

◆ Keep your immediate goals simple. Taking one step at a time is better than five one day and none the next.

MYTH: Exercising for 30 minutes two to three times per week is sufficient for weight loss.
FACT: That's better than doing nothing but it's not optimal. Our bodies are designed to be active daily. When we exercise daily we are healthier, leaner, more energetic – the list goes on and on.

READY, STEADY, GO!

11

Exercise intensity

Today, we're going to look at how to exercise at the right intensity (or heart rate zone), which is key to meeting your fitness goals.

First, you need to determine your maximum heart rate (MaxHR). There are two ways of doing this.

1. **Treadmill test** Undertaken in the company of a cardiologist or qualified exercise physiologist, this is the preferred method if you are over 40 years old. If you are overweight or have a family history of heart disease it is essential that you consult a cardiologist.
2. **Formula** If you have a sedentary lifestyle:
   220 minus your age
   If you exercise aerobically 3 or more time a week:
   205 minus your age

The heart rate zone at which you should exercise is also related to your personal fitness goal.

◆ If you are a beginner, with the goal of getting active, improving overall fitness or losing weight, you should be aiming to exercise in the **healthy heart zone** – 50–59% of your MaxHR.
◆ If you already exercise regularly and would like to lose body fat, exercise in the **fat-burning zone** – 60–69% of your MaxHR.
◆ If your goal is to improve aerobic capacity or athletic performance, exercise in the **aerobic zone** – 70–85% of your MaxHR.

The target zone chart in Appendix 3 will help you work out what your heart rate should be when exercising.

During exercise, briefly stop and locate your pulse. Once you've found it, begin counting each beat over a 15-second period – remember to use zero as your first count. Compare your pulse count with your target range, and you'll know right away if you're working out at your desired training level.

TOP TIP

- Keep temptation at bay when you're at home. Don't buy high-fat snacks such as nuts, crisps or mince pies if you can help it.
- If snacks have to be in your house keep them out of sight or store them in an awkward place so they're difficult to reach.

MYTH: Starving yourself is the best way to lose weight.
FACT: Starving yourself is the quickest way to get your body to lower its metabolism and energy levels – and bring your weight loss efforts to a screeching halt.

Activity

Active rest day

Active rest simply means moving around more than usual without actually doing a structured cardio workout. Whenever you get an opportunity to move, just make sure you do it – get off one bus or train stop earlier than usual, take the stairs, go and talk to someone rather than e-mailing them when at the office, walk the dog, walk to the shops, play with your children, rake the garden. If you sit all day, set an alarm to go off every hour and stand up and do some stretching. Be as active as you can. More activity equals a greater number of calories burned resulting in fat and weight loss!

READY, STEADY, GO!

13

Stay flexible

Make sure you spend a few minutes warming up before you stretch as you'll injure cold muscles more easily. March on the spot or walk up and down the stairs several times – or even have a hot bath to warm you up.

Do this stretching workout whenever you feel like it. Invest some quality time in de-stressing and unwinding with your stretches. Feel your body relaxing and all of the tension flowing out of the muscles then renewed energy flowing in.

Activity

Flexibility test

Today, we're assessing your current level of flexibility. You won't believe the difference the next few weeks will make! Next time we do this test, you will have improved dramatically – so make a note of today's results in your notebook.

Flexibility test

Sit and reach (testing back of thighs and hips)

1. Sit with your legs extended and feet flexed.
2. Keep your back straight, chest lifted, head in line with your spine and stomach in.
3. Look forward. Keeping your arms straight, breathe in as you reach skyward. Lead with your fingertips, then breathe out as you slowly and smoothly bend forwards from your hips.
4. Keep your back flat as you reach for your toes and don't crane your neck to try to reach further.

How did you get on?

- Finger extends past toes 2.5cm (one inch) or more – GOOD
- Finger reaches or almost reaches toes – AVERAGE
- Finger more than 12.5cm (5 inches) from toes – POOR

Shoulder extension (testing back of arms)

1. Breathe normally throughout.
2. Stand with your back straight, stomach muscles in and pelvis forward.
3. Bend your knees slightly. Reach up with your right arm, bend the elbow and drop your hand over your shoulder. Bend your left arm at the elbow and reach up behind your back. Slowly move your hands towards each other. Try to make your fingertips meet.

How did you get on?

- You can interlock your fingers – GOOD
- Fingertips touch – AVERAGE
- Finger more than 7.5cm (3 inches) apart – POOR

Forward flexion (testing lower back)

1. Sit with your back straight, chest lifted and stomach muscles in.
2. Extend your legs to the sides in a comfortable 'V'. Breathe in.
3. Breathe out as you slowly lean forward from your hips and lower back, and place your fists on the floor one on top of the other, between your legs.
4. Lower your chest toward your fists. Stop when you feel mild tension.
5. Measure the distance from the top of your top fist to your chest.

How did you get on?

- Chest at least 2.5cm (one inch) lower than fist – GOOD
- Chest reaches fist or within 5cm (2 inches) – AVERAGE
- Chest more than 30cm (12 inches) from fist – POOR

If your results weren't great, work a little harder on your stretching exercises to improve your rating when you try the test again.

READY, STEADY, GO!

Tone and strengthen

Resistance training

Resistance training uses resistance against body movements in order to tone and strengthen the muscles. You can use dumbbells, commercial weight machines, dyna-bands or surgical tubing, isometric exercises with a Swiss ball (also known as a fitness ball or thera-ball) or simple movements like curl ups, pull ups, push ups or squats. Resistance training:

◆ Increases metabolism by increasing lean muscle mass
◆ Increases bone density (which helps to decrease the chances of osteoporosis)
◆ Decreases the chance of joint injury
◆ Burns calories.

Do it twice a week or more and try to combine it with aerobic exercise. If you're a woman, don't worry about turning into a bodybuilder – even if you use heavy weights, your natural testosterone levels are too low to bulk you up beyond recognition.

Before you do today's activity, study the exercises in Appendix 1 to learn about the full range of resistance exercises in the *Body Idol* programme. If you have a dummy run, warm up first. For the real thing, work at a steady and controlled pace. Avoid rushing your exercises and if they become too hard to finish, then rest, as you don't want to injure yourself.

Sets and reps

A **repetition** (or **rep**) is one complete, single movement of a particular exercise.

A **set** represents a complete series or a set of exercises.

'Walking is the best possible exercise.' Thomas Jefferson,
3rd President of the United States

Activity
Toning and strength

Today marks the beginning of your stomach going from fat to flat. Strong, toned abdominal muscles not only contribute to good posture, but help keep your lower back free from aches and pains.

Make a real effort during your warm-up walk by striding out. Place your feet rather than stamping them down. Your breathing rate and body temperature should increase slightly. This means your work rate is about right. As you walk, plan other routes you'll want to try later in the week. (See Appendix 1 for the main exercises – their purpose and the technique.)

1. Cardio 8-minute power walk
2. Pelvic tilts: 1 set of 10 reps
3. Wall press ups: 1 set of 10 reps

Cool down with a sequence of stretches.

TOP TIP

◆ Set realistic goals. Having clear objectives and a challenging, yet achievable goal – such as losing three kilos before you go on holiday – will motivate you. Try signing a contract with yourself stating your goals.

MYTH: Now that I'm exercising, I can eat whatever I want.
FACT: Now that you're exercising, what you eat is even more important! You need your nutrients (not empty calories from fat and sugars) to fuel your body during exercise. You'll also feel more energised throughout the day, *not* just during exercise. You'll sleep better at night too and be able to fight off colds and infections better.

READY, STEADY, GO!

Your notes

CHAPTER 3

FOOD FACTS

Five-week 'kick start' healthy eating plan

To help you get the most of your new lifestyle programme, here's a sensible eating plan to set you on the road to healthier eating. Follow these recommended eating plans alongside your exercise programme for five weeks and you'll feel and see some dynamic results. After the fifth week, use what you have learned to compile your own eating plans in your notebook.

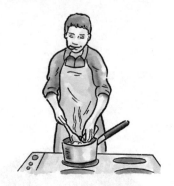

These tasty, easy-to-prepare meals are highly nutritious and you'll soon discover that healthy eating really isn't rocket science. If there are meal suggestions that don't suit your taste buds, reuse one of the light meal or main meal suggestions. Don't just stick to one or two – aim to eat a variety of the suggested meals as this will help you stick to the eating plan.

Allowances/recommendations

Water

It's vital that you drink at least one-and-a-half litres of water every day. This could be fizzy or still, plain or flavoured. This will ensure your body is kept hydrated, particularly if you lead a busy life with a fair degree of physical activity – and especially now that you've started an exercise programme.

Fruit/vegetables

Eat at least five portions of fruit and vegetables daily. One portion is equivalent to one apple. Aim for fresh produce and thoroughly wash or peel the outer skins before you eat.

Milk

Aim to drink or cook with at least a pint of skimmed, semi-skimmed milk, soya or goats milk every day.

FOOD FACTS

Extra virgin olive oil

Some of the menu suggestions will involve cooking with oil and some meals will include spreads on sandwiches. Always choose extra virgin olive oil for both of these as it's monounsaturated. This means that it helps to lower LDL cholesterol levels, without lowering high-density lipoprotein (HDL), the so-called 'good' cholesterol. (See Day 29 for more details about oils.)

Coffee and other hot drinks

Avoid coffee at all costs. Weak English or Indian tea is fine. Better still, drink fruit or herbal teas.

Fizzy/sugary drinks

Avoid these and substitute with water or freshly squeezed fruit juices.

Sugar

If you absolutely have to, use up to one dessert spoonful or three teaspoonfuls of sugar a day. If you normally use more than this throughout the day in tea/coffee or on breakfast cereal, either cut down or use an artificial sweetener instead.

Alcohol

You can enjoy up to four units of alcohol a week. One unit is equivalent to a half a pint of beer, one medium glass of wine or one measure of spirits. This quota may seem like very little, especially if you intend to go out for a few nights a week, but if you want to feel energised, four units is all you're allowed.

FOOD FACTS

Breakfast

The choices suggested below are suitable for everyone, whether you sit down to breakfast, eat on the go or eat breakfast at your desk. So, there's no excuse to skip it. After all, breakfast is the most important meal of the day and if you start without it, you're more likely to snack on high-calorie or high-fat foods later on in the day. Try mixing up the breakfast ideas at weekends when you can probably spend a little extra time in the kitchen.

Choose one of the following breakfast suggestions every day. Each option contains 280–300 calories.

◆ Medium bowl of cereal with milk
 One slice of wholemeal soda bread with marmalade/jam
 One small glass (100ml) of unsweetened orange, apple or cranberry juice.
 Choose this option for at least three days this week but avoid frosted/sugar-coated cereal.
◆ Cereal bar
 Apple/orange/three satsumas/one small banana
 One small carton of fruit juice (200ml)
◆ Fruit scone with olive oil-based spread and jam
 Tea
◆ Two slices of wholemeal soda bread with butter and a small banana
 Tea
◆ Three pancakes with maple syrup
 Tea

Mid-morning/mid-afternoon snack

Choose one of the following snacks for each day. It doesn't matter whether you have it at 10am, 3pm or 10pm but it makes sense to choose a time when you think you'll enjoy it most. For example, if you start work at 8am and don't have lunch until 1pm, mid-morning is probably the best time to have your snack. If you normally work late and don't have dinner until late evening, a mid-afternoon snack will keep you going.

FOOD FACTS

Each snack contains 60–100 calories.

- One wholemeal digestive biscuit
- Two chocolate chip cookies
- One small banana
- One apple
- Two fig rolls
- Diet fruit yoghurt
- Four rice cakes

Lunch/light meal

If it suits you to eat your main meal at lunch time or if, for example, you're going out to a restaurant for lunch, skip forward to the main meal section for suggestions. It doesn't make any difference to your diet whether you eat your main meal in the evening or at lunch time. But, it's important to eat something at lunch time to prevent snacking on high-calorie foods later on in the day.

The options listed below each contain between 400–450 calories.

Sandwiches

Enjoy a sandwich for lunch for five days this week. Choose your filling from the following suggestions.

- Low-fat cream cheese with oven-roasted peppers on granary bread (two slices)
  Fresh fruit
  Tea/mineral water/diet drink
- *Smoked salmon open sandwich on wholemeal soda bread (two slices) with a green salad and lemon wedge
  Fresh fruit
  Tea/mineral water/fruit juice
- *Tuna, sweetcorn and lettuce on wholegrain sliced bread (two slices)
  Fresh fruit
  Tea/mineral water/fruit juice

FOOD FACTS

23

- Brie and tomato relish open sandwich made with two slices of wholemeal soda bread, one triangle/30g brie and two teaspoonfuls of relish
  Fresh fruit
  Tea/mineral water/fruit juice
- Chicken tikka breast with iceberg lettuce on ciabatta bread
  Fresh fruit
  Tea/mineral water/fruit juice

★ Choose either low-fat mayonnaise or olive oil-based spread on your bread for these sandwiches, but not both. For all other sandwich suggestions, avoid salad dressing and butter.

Tip

Avoid baguette sandwiches as they're the equivalent of five slices of bread! For variety, go for flavoured, granary, rye or wholemeal soda bread, as well as sliced white bread.

Salads

- Caesar salad without croutons (ask for the salad dressing to be served on the side and use no more than two dessert spoonfuls of caesar dressing)
  One slice of wholemeal bread
  Fresh fruit
  Tea/mineral water/fruit juice
- Turkey and ham salad (one slice of turkey and one slice of ham) with green salad
  One dessert spoonful of pesto sauce and one dessert spoonful of flavoured oil as a dressing
  Fresh fruit
  Tea/mineral water/fruit juice

Main meal

You may choose to eat this meal earlier in the day and have a light meal from the lunch menu later – it's up to you.

FOOD FACTS

The main meal suggestions below contain 450–600 calories.

◆ *Pasta with tomato and ready-to-serve chilli sauce and large green salad*
Allow five handfuls of dried uncooked pasta per portion and enjoy one dessert spoonful of flavoured salad dressing oil on the salad. Avoid cream-based pasta sauces!

◆ *Spaghetti bolognaise*
Use three dessert spoonfuls of bolognaise, made from good-quality mince, per portion. Don't add any oil to the mince when frying. Serve with lots of spaghetti.

◆ *Chicken fajitas*
Use two flour tortillas per portion, filled with chicken, onion, lettuce, peppers, chilli and garlic. Fry the chicken in one-calorie spray oil. Add a tin of tomatoes when cooking all the other ingredients.

◆ *Beef or chicken curry and basmati rice*
Use 55–85g cooked weight of lean beef or one small chicken fillet and half a cup of uncooked rice per portion. Try to use homemade curry as this keeps the calories down. Don't add cream or coconut milk as both are high in fat and calories.

◆ *Stir-fry fish*
Stir-fry six prawns or six crab claws in olive oil, and add onions and carrots. Add three dessert spoonfuls of readymade sweet chilli sauce at the end of cooking. Serve with rice and a side salad.

◆ *Omelette*
Made with two eggs, fry with a knob of butter and fill with onion, tomato and 15g grated cheddar. Serve with a side salad.

◆ *Roast dinner of dry roast chicken, beef, lamb or pork*
Serve with two boiled potatoes and two fresh or frozen vegetables. Make gravy from granules rather than the juice of the meat as this can contain a lot of fat.

Note – side salad

Use a combination of all or some of the following: lettuce (all types), rocket, cucumber, peppers, tomatoes, but no dressing unless stated.

FOOD FACTS

Eat to live – not live to eat

What you eat plays a major role in how well you feel and how much energy you have. Food is the fuel that runs your body but it's also your body's building blocks. When you overeat, the extra food is stored as fat. When you exercise, the food is transformed into increasing your lean tissue.

You are what you eat

Today, good nutrition is more important than ever. Heart disease, cancer, stroke and diabetes are directly related to what we eat. Diet is also implicated in lots of other conditions.

Of course, food alone isn't the key to a longer and healthier life. Good nutrition should be part of a healthy lifestyle, which includes regular exercise, not smoking or drinking alcohol excessively, managing stress and limiting exposure to environmental hazards such as pollution. And, no matter how well you eat, your genes can affect how likely you are to get certain health problems. However, don't underestimate the influence of what you eat and how you eat it.

For example, atherosclerosis (hardening of the arteries) can begin in early childhood, but the process can be halted, even reversed, if you make healthy changes to your diet and lifestyle. You can slow gradual bone thinning that results in osteoporosis if your diet is rich in calcium, you get enough Vitamin D and you exercise regularly. Your genes may put you at risk of diabetes, but keep your weight within a healthy range through diet and exercise and the disease may never affect you.

FOOD FACTS

Balance, variety and moderation

To stay healthy, your body needs the right balance of carbohydrates, fats and protein. You also need vitamins, minerals and other goodies from many different foods. So, although some foods are better than others, no single food or food group has it all – so variety really is the spice of life.

Too much food can result in excess weight and even too much of certain nutrients, while eating too little can lead to numerous nutrient deficiencies and low body mass. Later on in this book, you'll gradually learn more about good nutrition

Activity

Cardio 9-minute power walk

Today we'll try another walking activity – 9 minutes this time. Remember to keep your head high and chest line out so that the muscles that help you breathe better can function properly and your lungs can expand as they take in oxygen. Enjoy breathing! Be conscious of breathing in and out.

After your invigorating walk, stretch out those muscles (see Appendix 1 for details of stretches). Why not spend a little longer holding every stretch? This will promote an even greater degree of flexibility and muscle tone.

TOP TIP

♦ When the going's getting tough, visualise the body you want to achieve – how you really want to look in your bikini or swimming trunks. That will make all your effort worthwhile.

FOOD FACTS

Carbohydrates

All foods provide differing amounts of carbohydrates, proteins, fats, vitamins, minerals, fibre and water.

Carbohydrates are the body's main source of energy and should be the major part of what we eat every day. They also provide your brain with energy, which is why a low-carb diet can make you feel 'spaced out'. All carbohydrates have roughly four calories a gram. Too many calories from carbohydrates at any one time will be stored as fat.

Complex carbs

These carbs, which are digested more slowly by the body, are less likely to be stored as fat and tend to be high in dietary fibre. These slow-burners include:

+ Oatmeal, wholegrain bread, grains, potatoes
+ Vegetables (mainly used as a source of fibre, vitamins and minerals, and not as a source of energy)
+ Pasta and rice – eat brown rice, which burns more slowly than white rice.

Complex carbohydrates are nutritious but have fewer calories per gram compared to fat. Eat some of these carbs before exercising to give you energy. Carbohydrates affect blood sugar, muscle glycogen levels and insulin production. Complex carbohydrates are good for diabetics because they allow better blood glucose control than simple carbs.

Simple carbs

Fast-burning carbohydrates (called sugars, simple carbs or simple sugars) are more likely to be stored as fat because the body doesn't get enough time to burn the calories.

These fast-burners include:

◆ Sweets
◆ Junk food containing sugar – biscuits, cakes, fizzy sugary drinks
◆ Fruit juice – not as good as fruit, but a better choice than junk food
◆ Fruit – still a very good source of fibre, vitamins and minerals.

When you eat simple carbs, your blood sugar increases relatively fast and then drops quickly, which will leave you feeling tired, sleepy and craving sugar or carbs even more. So avoid!

> **MYTH:** Carbohydrates make you fat.
> **FACT:** People have somehow got it in their heads that weight gain is all about the carbs, not the calories. People who quote this myth won't touch a potato (100 calories, 0g fat), but then will eat a 450g steak for dinner (915 calories, 57g fat). They'll refuse the hamburger bun (120 calories, 2g fat) but take an extra burger to make up for it (500 calories, 32g fat). The calorie counts say it all for this dieting myth. Some people on low-carb diets do lose weight initially, but this is mostly due to water and lean muscle loss, not fat loss. Overdosing on protein and cutting out carbs doesn't equal successful weight loss. What it does mean is missing out on vital nutrients from healthy carbohydrate foods that should be part of any well-balanced diet. If you're considering a low-carb diet, remember to count your calories and nutrients first.

Activity **Stretching exercises**

Ease yourself into every stretch (see the exercises in Appendix 1). Visualise your muscles relaxing and stretching further. Spend longer with every stretch. Why not perform every stretch twice?

FOOD FACTS

Proteins

Protein is the essential building block of muscle – without it, you can't and won't grow. Protein supplies amino acids to build and maintain healthy body tissue. Your body needs 20 essential amino acids in the right quantities to function properly – eight have to come from your diet.

Aim for a minimum of two grams of protein per kilo of bodyweight every day. All protein has roughly four calories a gram. Remember that your body will use protein as a source of energy instead of using it to build muscle if you're not getting enough calories from carbohydrates and dietary fats. This will rob you of good muscle tone and lean tissue, so eat enough quality carbs and fats too!

Protein sources include:

◆ All meat – including beef, poultry and fish
◆ All dairy products, including milk, cheese (high in fat!) and yoghurts
◆ Soya – all products
◆ Legumes (includes peanuts, soya beans)
◆ Nuts – a good way to add protein and healthy fats.

MYTH: Extra protein makes you strong.
FACT: The body has tremendous reserves and is very adaptable. The idea that you have to eat specific foods in specific amounts every day to maintain performance is unsound. When we're active, our body uses its own fat and carbohydrate for fuel. A diet that includes animal and vegetable protein supplies all that the body needs to replenish its stores. There is no super diet for super performance. Besides, high-protein diets often lack key nutrients found in carbohydrate foods. You need every kind of food – avoiding any kind of food is just as bad for you as taking food supplements.

FOOD FACTS

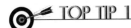

TOP TIP 1

◆ Remember, eat before you meet! Have a small meal before you go to any party like a hardboiled egg, apple and a thirst quencher (water, fruit juice, tea). This will help you cut down on the amount of alcohol you drink.

TOP TIP 2

◆ Stick to your fitness goals by thinking of them as promises to yourself, rather than as tests of your willpower.

Activity

Warm-up exercises/toning and strength

It's time to get your muscles even firmer and more taut. There's a great leg and buttock shaper at the end of this session – the half squat. (See main exercises in Appendix 1.)

1. Warm-up stretches
2. Wall press ups: 1 set of 11 reps
3. Pelvic tilts: 1 set of 11 reps
4. Half leg squats: 1 set of 10 reps

Cool down with a sequence of stretches focusing on your chest, stomach and legs.

FOOD FACTS

Fats

Fat supplies energy and transports nutrients. Fats, like carbohydrates, can either be burnt as energy or stored as body fat. Fats generally burn faster than carbs, so are more easily stored as body fat. Fats have roughly nine calories a gram. There's more info about fats in Day 29.

'Healthy' monounsaturated fats

'Healthy' fats provide a host of benefits, including giving you energy, maintaining overall health and making your skin and hair look better. Sources include:

◆ Fish oil (fats found in fish)
◆ Nuts (good source of protein and healthy fats)
◆ Olive oil
◆ Flaxseed oil – Essential Fatty Acids (EFAs).

Unhealthy saturated fats

'Unhealthy' fats (saturated fats) can drain you and affect your hair and skin. Sources include:

◆ Pastries, cakes and lots of ready meals
◆ Any deep-fried food (chips, fried chicken)
◆ Fat from animal sources, such as the saturated fats found in beef, pork and milk.

TOP TIP 1

• Save cash by taking a packed lunch to work. You need to be organised to do this, but it can be much cheaper than going to the sandwich shop every day. It's healthier, too, because you've got more control over what goes into your lunch.

FOOD FACTS

'Success is that old ABC – ability, breaks and courage.'
Charles Luckman, American architect and industrialist

TOP TIP 2

◆ Don't feel bad if you don't notice body changes right
away. It's only natural and we all experience this. Don't
forget – all good things come to those who wait!

MYTH: Everybody's resting heart rate is similar.
FACT: An average person's heart at rest beats
approximately 72 times a minute, while a fit
individual's resting heart rate is only around 55
beats a minute. That's a saving of 1,020 beats a
hour, 24,480 beats in 24 hours and 8,910,720
beats saved a year. If you got a similar saving on
petrol a year, you'd be running a car on peanuts!

Activity
Cardio 10-minute power walk

Start walking at a comfortable pace. Keep your
ears centred over your shoulders, which should be
centred over your hips. Don't slump. Keep your
chest up and out and your shoulders relaxed.
Always land on your heel first, rock, then swing
the foot forward. Keep your foot swing natural.
Don't forget to swing your arms!

After your workout, it's time to stretch. Do a quad
stretch, hamstring stretch, calf stretch and upper
back stretch, holding each for 30 seconds.

FOOD FACTS

Are you keeping up? Do you need some help? If you've not already subscribed, why not try the daily text messaging service for extra encouragement and support.
Just text 'Body Idol 11' to 80881 now.

Each set of messages costs £1.50. Please see page xiv for full terms and conditions.

Vitamins and minerals

Vitamins

Vitamins are found in food and are needed by the body in tiny amounts to regulate metabolism and maintain healthy growth and functioning. The most commonly known vitamins are A, B1 (thiamine), B2 (riboflavin), B3 (niacin), B5 (pantothenic acid), B6 (pyridoxine), B7 (biotin), B9 (folic acid), B12 (cobalamin), C (ascorbic acid), D, E and K. The B and C vitamins are water-soluble and excess amounts are passed in urine. The A, D, E and K vitamins are fat-soluble and will be stored in body fat.

Minerals

Minerals, for example, iron, calcium, phosphorus and chromium, are vital because they're the building blocks that make up muscles, tissues and bones. They're also important components of many life-supporting systems, such as hormones, oxygen transport and enzyme systems.

See the table in Appendix 4 for a detailed list of the best food sources for vitamins and minerals.

FOOD FACTS

TOP TIP 1

◆ Typical restaurant servings are often twice the size of a single serving. When eating out or getting a take-away, ask for half a serving or a doggy bag. That way, you won't be as full, and you can save some for tomorrow.

TOP TIP 2

◆ Don't worry about not having a fully equipped gym at home. Instead of lamenting what you don't have, find ways to make better use of what you do have!

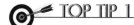

Active rest day

Don't just sit there – get up and do something! Try:

● Marching on the spot 100 times
● Walking up and down stairs 10 times
● Walking to the shops
● Cleaning the floors at home.

MYTH: The older you are, the less exercise you need.
FACT: As we get older our needs for specific types of exercise may change. A person may want to focus more on balance work such as yoga rather than a full-on aerobics workout or step class!

FOOD FACTS

Fibre and water

To broaden your knowledge even further on basic nutrition, here's the final instalment.

Fibre

This is the material that gives plants texture and support. Although it's primarily made up of carbohydrates, it doesn't have many calories and isn't usually broken down by the body for energy. It's partially digested in the stomach and intestines. Dietary fibre is found in plant foods such as fruit, vegetables, nuts and whole grains. There are two types of fibre: soluble and insoluble.

Soluble fibre

- It dissolves in water.
- It's found in a variety of fruit and vegetables such as apples, oatmeal and oat bran, rye flour and dried beans.
- It can lower blood cholesterol levels. It attaches itself to the cholesterol so that it can be eliminated from the body. This prevents cholesterol from re-circulating and being reabsorbed into the bloodstream.

Insoluble fibre

- It doesn't dissolve in water because it contains a large amount of cellulose.
- It's found in the bran of grains, fruit pulp and vegetable skin.
- It speeds up the transit of foods through the digestive system and adds bulk to the stools, and so helps with constipation or diarrhoea, and prevents colon cancer.

Water

You can last weeks without food, but without water, you'll curl your toes in a matter of days. Your body is about 70% water, so you can see how important it is. Water also helps to regulate body temperature, transports nutrients to cells and rids the body of waste materials.

FOOD FACTS

That's it – basic nutrition in a nutshell! All this interesting information makes you want to reach for a stick of celery!

TOP TIP

♦ Never focus on kilos – put away your scales and focus on eating sensibly.

MYTH: While light exercise does yield some benefits, it's not nearly as beneficial as strenuous exercise.
FACT: Strenuous workouts do improve aerobic capacity far more than light or moderate workouts. But while that may improve athletic performance, they don't necessarily translate into great health advantages. The death rates from coronary heart disease and cancer are much lower in moderate exercisers than in non exercisers – but they're only a little lower in heavy exercisers than in moderate exercisers. The same is true for the risk of developing type two diabetes (the most common kind). Non-strenuous exercise reduces stress, anxiety and blood pressure as effectively as strenuous exercise. And moderate exercise like walking can control weight just as effectively as vigorous exercise like jogging, since the calories you burn depends on how far you go, not how fast. In fact, moderate exercise is potentially more effective than vigorous exercise for most people, since they can walk much further than they can jog or run!

Activity
Stretching exercises

Your body should now be un-sticking itself! To further improve your range of movement, go and find a peaceful place and start stretching now! With each stretch, let the tension and stress eek out of those muscles.

FOOD FACTS

Good foods to eat

Natural states

The closer a food is to its natural state, the better it is for you. Fresh fruit and berries are packed with vitamins and will satisfy any craving for sweets. Green, orange and yellow vegetables have lots of vitamins and minerals too. Steam them to retain the most nutritional value. Be careful with sauces as they may be high in calories and fats that aren't good for you.

Go for wholegrain pasta

Avoid white bread and noodles because they're made from flour that has had much of the nutritional content removed. Also, the high starch content will affect your blood sugar as quickly as regular sugar. Avoid sugary snacks and pastries too.

Shop for lean meats and don't forget the fish

Our diets are often lacking in omega three oils, which are found ocean fish, so serve seafood two or three times a week. Fish and chicken is healthier grilled or baked rather than fried, and lean meats like venison are healthier than higher-fat beef. Processed meats, hot dogs, bacon and sausages have a lot of junk in them, but if you love them, aim for healthier organic versions, which are increasingly available in supermarkets and local butchers.

Eat a variety of foods

One good reason to do this is that some people become sensitive to foods they eat frequently. Try different grains as a substitute for wheat, and try rice milk or soya milk instead of cow's milk. Experiment with new foods even if you think you won't like them – it can be a lot of fun and great on the taste buds.

Stick to water

Aim to consume water as your main drink and avoid fizzy drinks (both sugary and diet). If you get tired of water, add a slice of lemon or lime. You could also jazz up some fruit juice with sparkling water. Some herbal and green teas are good for you, but avoid too much caffeine.

'Do what you can, with what you have, where you are.'
Theodore Roosevelt, 26th President of the United States

TOP TIP

♦ Make your workout weather-proof. Get the right workout gear so weather conditions are never an excuse.

Activity
Cardio 11-minute walk

You may be a little sore after the last few days' exercises, but don't worry. This will soon go. You'll feel much better from your effort and lifestyle changes. Today, walk slightly faster and more upright than you're used to. It may be a bit difficult, but hang in there. Regulate your breathing and make sure you lead with your heel and roll through to the ball of your foot.

After your walk, spend some time stretching out your muscles, with a particular emphasis on your leg muscles.

FOOD FACTS

Your notes

....

....

....

....

....

....

....

....

....

....

....

....

....

....

....

....

....

....

....

....

....

....

CHAPTER 21

SLEEP IS FOR LIVING, SMOKING IS FOR GIVING UP

How did you get on with Week 1 of your healthy eating plan? You're sure to have shed the odd kilo already. The basis of your kick-start eating plan was to help you identify what foods are healthy and nutritious and for you to realise how tasty and easy these foods are to prepare. You're now ready for Week 2!

Breakfast

Choose one of the following breakfast suggestions every day. Each option contains 280–300 calories.

- ◆ Medium bowl of cereal with milk
  One slice of wholemeal soda bread or toast with jam/marmalade
  Small glass of unsweetened or fresh fruit juice (100ml)
  Choose this option on at least four days this week.
- ◆ Two slices of toast with one poached/scrambled egg
  One grilled tomato
  One small glass (100ml) of orange juice
- ◆ Large bowl of fresh fruit salad
  Fruit yoghurt
  Large glass water
- ◆ Porridge/toasted oat cereal made with milk, not hot water

Mid-morning/mid-afternoon snack

Choose one of the following snacks each day. It doesn't matter whether you have it at 10am, 3pm or 10pm but it makes sense to choose a time when you think you'll enjoy it most. For example, if you start work at 8am and don't have lunch until 1pm, mid-morning is probably the best time to have your snack. If you normally work late and don't have dinner until late evening, a mid-afternoon snack will keep you going.

Each snack contains 60–100 calories.

- ◆ One diet yoghurt
- ◆ Six marshmallows
- ◆ Slice of toast with olive-oil spread/jam/marmalade

Lunch/light meal

If it suits you to eat your main meal at lunch time or if, for example, you're going out to a restaurant for lunch, skip forward to the main meal section for suggestions. It doesn't make any difference to your diet whether you eat your main meal in the evening or at lunch time. But, it's important to eat something at lunch time to prevent snacking on high-calorie foods later on in the day.

The options listed below each contain between 400–450 calories.

Sandwiches

Choose either low-fat mayonnaise or olive-oil spread but not both on your sandwich.

♦ Chicken, lettuce and sweetcorn sandwich on white sliced/ wholemeal bread using one small chicken fillet (50g cooked weight), 10g (two teaspoonfuls) low-fat mayonnaise, lettuce, sweetcorn
Fruit
Fruit juice/mineral water/tea

♦ Ham and iceberg lettuce sandwich on wholemeal bread, using wafer-thin premium ham (one large slice) and iceberg lettuce
Fruit
Cappuccino (made using skimmed milk)/tea/flavoured mineral water

♦ Chicken curry wrap with lettuce and peppers using one small chicken fillet (50g cooked weight), 10g (two teaspoonfuls) low-fat curry mayonnaise, iceberg lettuce, peppers, one flour tortilla
Fruit
Fruit juice/mineral water/tea

♦ Cheddar cheese and chutney sandwich on wholemeal or white batch bread, using 50g grated low-fat cheddar, three teaspoonfuls (15g) chutney
Fruit
Fruit juice/mineral water/tea
Tip: Spread the chutney on the bread first and the grated cheese will stick to it. No need for butter or mayonnaise.

◆ Houmous with roasted peppers and lettuce in a pitta pocket using 100g low-calorie hummus, roasted peppers, iceberg lettuce, one pitta pocket (50g)
Fruit
Fruit juice/mineral water/tea

◆ Roasted peppers with salsa and sour cream in a wrap using roasted peppers, three dessert spoonfuls of salsa (homemade if possible), 10g (two teaspoonfuls) sour cream/crème fraiche or natural bio yoghurt, one flour tortilla
Fresh fruit
Cappuccino (made with skimmed milk)/flavoured mineral water/tea/fruit juice

Another lunch option

◆ A large bowl of low-fat vegetable soup
A boiled egg and one slice of wholemeal soda bread with olive-oil spread
Fresh fruit
Fruit juice/mineral water/tea

Main meal

You can choose to eat this meal earlier in the day and have a light meal from the lunch menu later – it's up to you.

The main meal suggestions below contain 450–600 calories.

◆ *Shepherd's pie and beans*
Use a good-quality lean mince and don't add oil during cooking – it will brown with gentle cooking without any added fat. Only use milk to mash the potatoes. Enjoy a 10cm square portion and freeze any leftovers.

◆ *Two large baked potatoes and filling*
Dry roast the potatoes on a salted baking tray on the top shelf of the oven. Filling suggestions: 30g grated Edam cheese or three dessert spoonfuls of chilli-con-carne/bolognaise sauce. Enjoy a small side salad with this meal.

◆ *Chicken casserole with rice or two medium-sized boiled potatoes*
Allow one medium-sized chicken fillet per portion and fry in olive oil with onions. Use a vegetable/chicken stock cube rather than soup or packet casserole mixes. Allow half a cup of uncooked rice per portion.

◆ *Stir-fry vegetables and rice*
Use any combination of vegetables, e.g. baby corn, mange tout, onions and peppers. Enjoy a generous amount as vegetables are very low in calories. Stir-fry in one teaspoonful of olive oil. Add two dessert spoonfuls of flavoured sauce such as sweet chilli or plum and sesame sauce at the end of cooking.

◆ *Chicken satay and rice*
Fry one medium-sized chicken fillet in one-calorie cooking oil spray. Coat the chicken with one dessert spoonful of ready made satay sauce at the end of cooking. Satay sauce is delicious and very high in calories so don't coat the chicken with more than the amount recommended. Serve the chicken on skewers or in strips with rice and a side salad.

◆ *Baked breaded fish fillet and baked potatoes*
Once a week, enjoy a 100g serving of breaded fish fillet baked in the oven. Serve with two medium-sized baked potatoes and two fresh or frozen vegetables.

◆ *Roast dinner of beef, lamb or pork*
Chicken has featured widely this week so go for a roasted meat dish. Choose two large slices of meat with two boiled potatoes and two fresh or frozen vegetables. Make gravy from granules or stock and not the juice from the meat as this contains a lot of fat and calories.

Tip

Vegetables are very low in calories as long as they're boiled, steamed or cooked in a very small amount of oil or butter (one teaspoonful or one knob) so you can eat lots of them. They're also a rich source of vitamins and minerals.

Note – side salad

Use a combination of all or some of the following: lettuce, all types, rocket, cucumber, peppers, tomatoes, but no dressing unless stated.

SLEEP IS FOR LIVING, SMOKING IS FOR GIVING UP

Assess your lifestyle

Once you've learnt about which foods are good for you, it's worth looking at your eating habits. If the foods you eat aren't healthy, it's best to try and work within your current habits and lifestyle, rather than making drastic changes. Consider these questions then, over the next few days, read on for tips to help you add healthy foods.

- Do you eat because you're bored, sad or happy?
- Do you snack in front of the TV without even giving it much thought?
- Do you eat most of your meals at home or in restaurants?
- How often do you eat fast food?
- Do you like to cook?
- How often do you grocery shop?
- Do you skip breakfast or lunch, then overeat later in the day?
- How big are the portions you eat?
- Do you crave sweets?
- Are there foods you refuse give up?

TOP TIP 1

- Just because something is called a salad, it doesn't mean it's good for you! Coleslaw, macaroni salad and potato salad usually contain lots of mayonnaise, which is high in fat and calories. One way to lighten the load is to dress these salads with low-fat mayonnaise, balsamic vinegar and yoghurt. Bulk things up by adding celery, onions and hard-boiled egg.

TOP TIP 2

- It's often hard to motivate yourself to eat healthily. Sometimes, you can't rely on motivation alone – you need to set up your environment to support healthy eating. One of the easiest ways to do this is to stop keeping 'naughty' foods at home. Out of sight, out of mind can be a huge help in healthy eating!

SLEEP IS FOR LIVING, SMOKING IS FOR GIVING UP

'A sound mind in a sound body is a thing to be prayed for.'
Juvenal, Roman writer

Activity

Toning and strength

You've been on this programme for over two weeks now. Well done! Achieving that highly toned and chiselled look takes real effort and with the combination of your toning exercises, you're well and truly on your way to a super-sleek body. Really work those muscles with these three new exercises. They're challenging, so keep an eye on your technique (see Appendix 1, main exercises).

1. Modified floor press ups: 1 set of 10 reps

2. Abdominal curls: 1 set of 10 reps

3. Half leg squats: 1 set of 10 reps

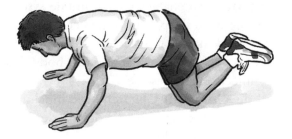

Unwind with some stretches afterwards.

MYTH: Low-carbohydrate diets such as the Atkins diet are a safe and effective way to lose weight. **FACT:** Low-carb diets may be harmful. What's more, the weight loss they produce appears to be the result of a reduction in overall calories, not just a reduction in carbohydrates.

SLEEP IS FOR LIVING, SMOKING IS FOR GIVING UP

Sound asleep

Sleep is one of your body's most mysterious, complicated processes, which even scientists don't fully understand. But what we do know is that sleep is essential for the normal, healthy functioning of the human body.

Sleep helps your body restore and rejuvenate in many different ways including:

◆ **Memory, learning and social processes** Sleep enables the brain to encode new information and store it properly. REM (rapid eye movement) sleep activates the parts of the brain that control learning. The parts of the brain that control emotions, decision-making and social interactions slow down dramatically during sleep, allowing optimal performance when awake.
◆ **Nervous system** Some sleep experts suggest that neurons used during the day repair themselves during sleep. When you're deprived of sleep, neurons can't perform effectively and the nervous system is impaired.
◆ **Immune system** Sleep enables your immune system to function effectively. During deep sleep, your body's cells increase production while proteins break down at a slower rate. Without proper sleep, your immune system weakens and your body becomes more vulnerable to infection and disease.
◆ **Growth and development** Children need much more sleep than adults. Growth hormones are released during sleep, so sleep is vital to physical and mental development.

Stages of sleep

Stage 1 is dozing. It's a period of very light sleep in which you're easily awakened. You may feel like you're falling and jerk suddenly awake – this is called a hypnic jerk.

Stage 2 – the majority of sleep is spent in this stage.

Stages 3 and 4 are very deep sleep. It's very difficult to wake you and you often feel groggy and disoriented for several minutes. REM sleep, which happens here, is often referred to as dream sleep. During this time, your brain blocks signals to your muscles so they stay immobile so you won't act out on your dreams.

How much sleep do I need?

Everybody's sleep requirement is different. The average adult functions best after seven to eight hours sleep, although the amount ranges from five to ten hours a night. Women in the first trimester of pregnancy, and sometimes throughout pregnancy, need significantly more sleep than usual.

Some of the signs that you might need more sleep include:

◆ Difficulty waking up in the morning
◆ Inability to concentrate, even on simple tasks
◆ Slow reactions and poor memory
◆ Falling asleep during work or class
◆ Feelings of moodiness, irritability, depression or anxiety
◆ Needing to drop off during the day.

Not getting enough sleep can cause a 'sleep debt', which your body expects to make up. Severe sleep deprivation can lead to physical incapacity, hallucinations and mood swings.

'The body of man or woman is a machine which winds its own springs.' J. O. De La Mettrie, French physician and philosopher

Activity

Active rest day

Decide on three chores around the office or at home that are physically active. Examples include using the stairs at work, clearing up your house or mowing the lawn. Anything extra you do on top is a bonus.

SLEEP IS FOR LIVING, SMOKING IS FOR GIVING UP

Insomnia

'The preservation of health is a duty. Few seem conscious that there is such a thing as physical morality.' Herbert Spencer, Victorian biologist and early social philosopher

What if I have trouble going to sleep? Is it insomnia?

Symptoms of insomnia include difficulty dropping off, waking frequently during the night or early morning, and not feeling refreshed. Although insomnia is most common in women and older adults, everyone can experience it. Over 90% of people in the UK have short-term insomnia at some point – this is often caused by a temporary situation, such as a relationship problem, work worries, a short illness or jet lag. Up to 30% of people struggle with chronic or long-term insomnia. This lasts for a month or more – sometimes years.

What causes insomnia?

- **Lifestyle factors** Alcohol and stimulants (i.e. caffeine, nicotine and non-prescription medications), erratic hours, changes in sleeping/waking (i.e. jet lag). See more below.
- **Environmental factors** Noise, light, extreme temperatures and changes in the surrounding environment.
- **Psychological disorders** Depression often causes insomnia, which has also been linked to other psychological disorders including anxiety, bipolar disorder and post-traumatic stress.
- **The menopause** Many women experiencing the menopause have insomnia. Hot flushes during sleep can induce a lighter, less restful and restorative stage of sleep.
- **Illness or medical problems** Common conditions that often cause or worsen insomnia include arthritis, chronic pain, breathing problems, heart conditions and hormonal or digestive disorders.
- **Sleep-related disorders** Circadian rhythm disorders, sleep apnoea, periodic limb movement or restless legs syndrome can cause insomnia.

Effects of caffeine, medications, heavy smoking and alcohol

Some foods and medicines alter the brain signals that control sleep and wakefulness. Which of these do you need to address?

- Caffeine (found in coffee, tea, cola and chocolate) is a stimulant. Try stopping your caffeine intake earlier in the day to ensure you get quality sleep.
- Eating spicy and acidic foods, or a big meal close to bedtime, can cause heartburn and indigestion. Eat lighter meals earlier and allow two to three hours to digest before bedtime.
- Herbal supplements and over-the-counter or prescription medications, such as diet pills, decongestants and energy-boosting supplements can disrupt sleep. Many antidepressants suppress REM sleep, leading to disrupted sleep cycles. Read labels carefully and consult your doctor if you're concerned.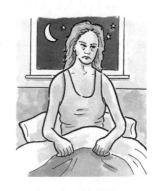
- Nicotine stimulates the brain. Regular smokers often sleep very lightly and have reduced amounts of REM sleep.
- Alcohol can induce a light sleep but impairs the more restorative stages of sleep. It prevents REM sleep and deeper sleep.

Activity

Cardio 12-minute power walk

Keep up a good pace so you feel slightly breathless – this encourages your body to use more energy and burn fat. Pump with those arms as you take long strides with your legs, softly landing on your heels first and following through onto the balls of your feet.

Don't forget your stretches afterwards!

SLEEP IS FOR LIVING, SMOKING IS FOR GIVING UP

A good night's sleep

Do you have trouble falling asleep? Or wake in the night and can't get back to sleep? If so, you're one of the million people who have some form of insomnia.

Tips for a better sleep environment

◆ Make sure your bed is large enough and comfortable. Test different types of mattresses. Try therapeutic-shaped foam pillows that cradle your neck or extra pillows that help you sleep on your side. Get comfortable cotton sheets.
◆ Make your bedroom primarily a place for sleeping. Try not to use your bed for paying bills, doing work, etc.
◆ Keep your bedroom peaceful and comfortable. Make sure your room is well ventilated and the temperature consistent. And try to keep it quiet.

Tips for a better pre-sleep ritual

◆ Try to go to bed and wake up at the same time every day, even on the weekends.
◆ Incorporate bedtime rituals. Listening to soft music, sipping a cup of herbal tea, etc. tells your body that it's time to slow down and prepare for sleep.
◆ Don't eat a large, heavy meal within two to three hours of going to bed.
◆ Bedtime snacks can help. Tryptophan, which is found in milk, turkey and peanuts, helps the brain produce serotonin, a chemical that helps you relax. Try drinking warm milk or eat a slice of toast or a bowl of cereal before bedtime.
◆ Jot down any worries. Anxiety excites the nervous system, so your brain sends messages to the adrenal glands, making you more alert.
◆ Go to sleep when you're sleepy.
◆ Avoid over-the-counter 'sleep aids' and make sure that any prescribed medication doesn't cause insomnia. There's little evidence that supplements and other sleep aids are effective.

SLEEP IS FOR LIVING, SMOKING IS FOR GIVING UP

Tips for getting back to sleep

◆ Visualise. Focus all your attention on your toes or visualise walking down an endless staircase. Thinking about mindless or repetitive things will help your brain shut down.

◆ Get out of bed if you can't sleep. Go into another room and do something relaxing until you feel sleepy.

◆ Don't do anything stimulating like watching a lively TV programme. Don't expose yourself to bright light, which tells your brain to wake up.

◆ Try changing your bedtime. Try going to bed later so that the time you spend in bed is spent sleeping. Once you start sleeping well, you can gradually sleep more, by adding 15 minutes at a time.

Activity

Mobility exercises/ toning and strength

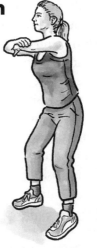

Today is sculpting day. Get your body warmed up and go for these super toners. Make sure you focus on good posture and technique – it's both quality and quantity that counts.

1. Modified floor press ups: 1 set of 12 reps

2. Abdominal curls: 1 set of 12 reps

3. Half leg squats: 1 set of 12 reps

Afterwards, why not spend a little longer holding every stretch? Not only will you add to your flexibility and muscle tone, but you can let go of the stresses of the day and clear any negative thoughts.

SLEEP IS FOR LIVING, SMOKING IS FOR GIVING UP

The more you puff it, the sooner you snuff it

Cigarette smoking is the number one preventable cause of death among men and women. Addiction to nicotine is the main factor in dependency on cigarettes. Nicotine causes a physiological 'rush' – an increase in blood pressure, breathing and heart rate caused by adrenaline. Nicotine can also have a sedative effect as it increases the levels of dopamine (the chemical that activates the parts of the brain controlling pleasure).

Top five health risks of smoking

1. The risk of a smoker aged 45–74 dying is more than double that of a non-smoker of the same age.
2. The risk of getting lung cancer increases with quantity, duration and intensity of smoking. A woman who smokes 40 or more cigarettes a day is 20 times more likely to die of lung cancer than a female non-smoker.
3. Women who stop smoking before or during pregnancy reduce the risk of reproductive problems, including infertility, premature birth and low birth weight.
4. Male smokers have a lower sperm count and a higher incidence of abnormal sperm compared to non-smokers. Sperm counts rise when a man stops smoking.
5. Exposure to environmental tobacco smoke can cause lung cancer in non-smokers and is associated with increased coronary heart disease risk.

And there's more…

Not yet convinced about the ill effects of smoking? Here are some more facts:

Starting at the top Smokers are at risk of mouth cancer. Tobacco smoke can also cause gum disease, tooth decay and bad breath. Smokers may get frequent headaches. Lack of oxygen and narrowed blood vessels to the brain can lead to strokes.

The lungs and breathing tubes Chemicals in smoke attack the lining of the breathing tubes, inflaming them and causing chronic smoker's cough. You're more likely to get bronchial infections and suffer from chronic coughing. Smokers are ten times more likely than non-smokers to get lung cancer and emphysema.

The heart Nicotine raises blood pressure and makes the blood clot more easily. Carbon monoxide robs the blood of oxygen and leads to cholesterol deposits developing on the artery walls. These all increase the risk of a heart attack. Also, the poor circulation from cholesterol deposits can cause strokes.

Other organs The tars in smoke can trigger cancer of the oesophagus and throat. Smoking causes increased stomach acid, leading to heartburn and ulcers. Smokers have higher rates of fatal pancreatic cancer. Many of the carcinogens from cigarettes come out in the urine where they can cause bladder cancer. High blood pressure from smoking can damage the kidneys.

Activity

Cardio 13-minute power walk

It really doesn't take long to build good habits into your daily routine. Your body will appreciate what you're doing – and you're making yourself feel good too! Keep walking at a pace that encourages you to breathe slightly more heavily, while at the same time increasing your body temperature.

During your stretching, spend some time reflecting on your achievements so far. Think only positive and constructive thoughts as you breathe in, and breathe away any negatives thoughts.

SLEEP IS FOR LIVING, SMOKING IS FOR GIVING UP

Top tips for giving up smoking

We all know smoking's bad for you – it doesn't make giving up any easier. But the long-term health risks just can't be ignored and it's never too late to say no to nicotine. Follow these tips for a life where you can breathe more easily.

1. **Professional support** Get as much help as possible from support organisations. There are plenty around and they've helped millions of smokers give up every year and have invaluable advice. National No Smoking Day, every March, is a good time to give up.
2. **With a little help from my friends** Enlist a fellow fagger in giving up. Give each other forfeits if you fail, rewards if you succeed and a shoulder to cry on when it all gets too tough.
3. **Body overhaul** Start an exercise and diet regime at the same time. Changing your lifestyle may initially seem like hell, but you'll see and feel the benefits in no time – and also avoid piling on those notorious giving-up-smoking kilos!
4. **Face facts** Visit a beautician to see the long-term damage smoking does to your skin. You'll be shocked by the premature ageing smoking can cause – worse even than exposure to the sun.
5. **Show me the money** Consider the cash you'll be saving by giving up. If you've got a 20-a-day habit, then you're spending nearly £40 a week. That's over £2,000 a year – or a brand-new wardrobe, a luxury Caribbean holiday, a state-of-the-art TV …

Withdrawal symptoms

Withdrawal can be extremely unpleasant and can include:

- Craving
- Difficulty thinking and concentrating
- Increased appetite
- Irritability
- Sleep disturbance.

Symptoms may start within a few hours of the last cigarette, peak within a few days and last from a few weeks to six months or more.

The results

You've stopped smoking and already your skin is healthier because it's getting more oxygen and blood – and is ageing more slowly than when you smoked. Your hands have lost that yellowish tint and your teeth aren't being stained any more. Plus your breath, hair and clothes no longer smell like an ashtray ...

When you give up smoking your body begins to repair itself. Ten years after you give up, your body has repaired most of the damage smoking caused.

Activity

Active rest day

While today's a rest day, it doesn't mean you can lie around and do nothing! Try some of these ideas:

- Set an alarm to go off every hour. Walk or stretch for five minutes.

- When it's break time at work, take a 10-minute walk up and down the stairs or around the building.

- When you get home from work, try a few stretches.

- If you're watching TV, do abdominal curls or press ups during the adverts.

SLEEP IS FOR LIVING, SMOKING IS FOR GIVING UP

Solutions for snackers

If you're an emotional eater or have an increased appetite due to giving up smoking, keep the junk food like crisps, tortilla chips, ice cream and sweets out of the house. Keep healthy snacks handy like fruit or crunchy vegetables with dips. If you really must have a treat, then buy a small piece of high-quality chocolate or your favourite treat and enjoy it. Just don't buy any to bring home!

The same tips are helpful for those who enjoy TV snacking at home. If you don't want to give up nibbling while glued to the box, keep low-calorie foods close by, because it's very easy to eat too much when you're caught up in your favourite programme.

Activity

Cardio 14-minute power walk

This point marks the end of another week and the start of a new week. This means challenges! Keep up the walking. By now you're walking with a spring in your step and bouncing with energy. Keep up a good pace and check your posture and technique. Swing your arms energetically like pistons pumping up and down, backward and forwards. You'll find this will help your momentum and rhythm.

Keep those limbs loose and supple, and avoid soreness by completing your stretches. Hold every one for as long as you can – time permitting.

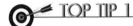

TOP TIP 1

♦ Stop adding salt to food. Too much salt can raise blood pressure and increase the risk of heart disease and strokes. Get into the habit of checking food labels, as many processed foods are high in salt. Adults should try to eat no more than 2.5g sodium (6g salt) a day.

TOP TIP 2

♦ Make household chores count. Mop the floor, scrub the bathtub or do other housework. Stretching and lifting is good exercise. Work at a fast pace to get your heart pumping. Try working in the garden as well, mowing the lawn or taking out weeds. Gardening can burn up to 300 calories an hour and is a great way to build strength. Raking and hoeing strengthen your arms and back, while digging works your arms and legs.

MYTH: A kilogram of fat is a kilogram of fat, regardless of where it is on the body.
FACT: Extra fat in your abdominal area is decidedly unhealthier than extra fat around your hips, buttocks and thighs. Research has shown that 'apple' shapes are at a greater risk of developing a number of health-related problems, the most common being hypertension, type two diabetes and hyperlipidemia (elevated levels of fat in the blood).

SLEEP IS FOR LIVING, SMOKING IS FOR GIVING UP

Your notes

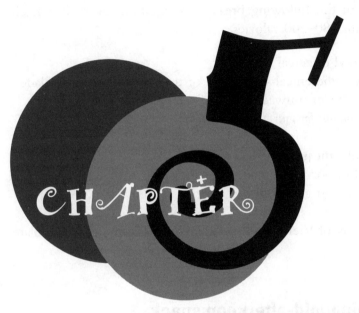

CHAPTER 5

FOOD FOR LIFE

Eating sensibly and healthily is as simple as A, B, C. You're now discovering that good, wholesome food can still be 'fancy' and healthy. Here's your Week 3 instalment – watch those kilos drop away!

Breakfast

Choose one of the following breakfast suggestions every day. Each option contains 280–300 calories.

- Medium bowl of cereal with milk
  One slice of wholemeal soda bread or toast with jam/marmalade
  One small glass of unsweetened or fresh fruit juice (100ml)
  Choose this option for four days this week.
- Muesli
  One glass of fruit juice (100ml)
- Large bowl of porridge (made with milk)
  One slice of toast and honey
  Tea
- Three rounds of Vienna/Kaiser roll white bread with chocolate spread
  Tea

Mid-morning/mid-afternoon snack

Choose one of the following snacks each day. It doesn't matter whether you have it at 10am, 3pm or 10pm but it makes sense to choose a time when you think you'll enjoy it most. For example, if you start work at 8am and don't have lunch until 1pm, mid-morning is probably the best time to have your snack. If you normally work late and don't have dinner until late evening, a mid-afternoon snack will keep you going.

Each snack contains 60–100 calories.

- Plain popcorn (small bag)
- Four satsumas
- Large bowl of soup (300ml) – go for the low-fat range

- Fruit smoothie drink, made with two small pieces of fruit
- One small slice of carrot cake
- Apple

Lunch/light meal

If it suits you to eat your main meal at lunch time or if, for example, you're going out to a restaurant for lunch, skip forward to the main meal section for suggestions. It doesn't make any difference to your diet whether you eat your main meal in the evening or at lunch time. But, it's important to eat something at lunch time to prevent snacking on high-calorie foods later on in the day.

The options listed below each contain 400–450 calories.

- One garlic pitta pocket filled with chicken tikka breast (50g) and iceberg lettuce
  Fresh fruit
  Cappuccino (skimmed milk)/tea
- ★Silverside corn beef sandwich with lettuce and tomato on white bread (two wafer-thin slices of silverside corn beef and not the processed corn beef)
  Fresh fruit
  Tea/flavoured mineral water
- Toasted cheese, tomato and onion sandwich (use 30g of Edam or low-fat cheddar if making at home)
  Fresh fruit salad
  Tea/fruit juice/mineral water
- ★Turkey sandwich with lettuce and cherry tomatoes on granary bread
  Fresh fruit
  Cappuccino/latte (skimmed milk)/tea
- ★Smoked salmon open sandwich on two slices of wholemeal soda bread, lemon wedge and capers
  Fresh fruit
  Tea/fruit juice or mineral water

FOOD FOR LIFE

- Large bowl of soup (no bread or roll)
  Two triangles of Irish cheese and redcurrant jelly
  One slice of wholemeal soda bread
  Tea/fruit juice/mineral water
- Egg salad sandwich on white/wholemeal bread
  Fresh fruit
  Cappuccino/latte (skimmed milk)/tea

* Choose either olive-oil spread or low-calorie mayonnaise on these sandwiches but not both.

Main meal

You can choose to eat this meal earlier in the day and have a light meal from the lunch menu later – it's up to you.

The main meal suggestions below contain 450–600 calories.

- *Pizza*
  Two small (75g each) cheese and tomato pizzas or two slices of pizza (150g total weight). Add low-calorie toppings such as onions, mushrooms and peppers. Enjoy with a side salad.

- *Pasta with chicken and pesto sauce*
  Allow three handfuls of dried uncooked pasta shapes per portion. Stir-fry a small chicken fillet that's been cut into thin strips in one-calorie cooking oil spray. Add two dessert spoonfuls of pesto sauce to the chicken and pasta.

- *Pasta and ratatouille*
  Allow five handfuls of dried uncooked pasta shapes a portion. Add a large portion of ratatouille (homemade if possible) to the cooked pasta and serve with 30g of Edam cheese grated on top.

FOOD FOR LIFE

◆ *Sausages and mash*

Two grilled sausages with two scoops of mashed potato (mash potatoes with milk only) and beans (small tin 141g). Sausages are very high in calories and so this meal will appear small on a plate – it might not be very filling either!

◆ *Stew*

Irish stew/beef casserole with two medium-sized boiled potatoes.

◆ *Burger and chips*

Homemade 100g beef burger and oven chips. Use good-quality lean mince to make the burger. Add seasoning and half a chopped onion to make the burger. Fry the onions and burger in olive oil and serve in a toasted bun with 100g (cooked weight) of sunflower oil oven chips (small portion). Enjoy with a side salad.

◆ *Roast dinner*

Roast dinner of turkey and ham, beef, lamb, pork or chicken. Two large slices of meat with two boiled potatoes and two fresh or frozen vegetables. Make gravy from granules or stock, not from meat juice, as this contains a lot of fat and calories.

Note – side salad

Use a combination of all or some of the following: lettuce (all types), rocket, scallions, cucumber, peppers, tomatoes, but no dressing unless stated.

FOOD FOR LIFE

Are you keeping up? Do you need some help? If you've not already subscribed, why not try the daily text messaging service for extra encouragement and support.
Just text 'Body Idol 21' to 80881 now.

Each set of messages costs £1.50. Please see page xiv for full terms and conditions.

Tips for eating out

Keep the portions small It can be really difficult to stay healthy if you eat out a lot... those salads might not be as appealing as a greasy cheeseburger and chips! Restaurants sometimes serve huge portions of food too. If you haven't got the willpower to stick to the salads – pick out a starter you love, combine it with a salad or a soup and skip the larger starters. You can also share a meal or take half of it home.

Dying for pud? Order as small a size as possible or perhaps just one scoop of ice cream, rather than a larger, heavier desert. Try a dish of mixed berries topped with nuts and a small portion of whipped cream.

Ration the red wine Be careful with the after-dinner drinks too. Perhaps have just one glass of wine with your meal. Drinking too much with your meal means you're more likely to overeat.

Skip the fast food If you eat a lot of fast food, you'll know how difficult it is to feel good and stay healthy. Some fast-food places have added salads and some better choices, but it really isn't a good way to eat. Keep fast-food dining to a minimum – don't go for the large sizes and choose places that offer more fresh ingredients.

> **MYTH:** Don't drink water unless you're thirsty.
> **FACT:** It's important to drink water or other fluids without caffeine before, during and after exercise. Take a water break even if you're not thirsty. You need to regularly replace the fluids you're losing when you exercise. Otherwise, you could become dehydrated to such an extent that it affects your performance and how you feel.

FOOD FOR LIFE

TOP TIP

◆ Eat more fish. White fish (such as haddock, plaice, halibut and sole) and oily fish (such as sardines, salmon, trout, pilchards and mackerel) are valuable sources of protein, vitamins and minerals. Aim to eat at least two servings of fish a week, including one portion of oily fish. Oily fish contains omega three polyunsaturated fatty acids, which can help prevent coronary heart disease.

'Health and intellect are the two blessings of life.' Menander, Greek playwright

Activity

Mobility exercises/ toning and strength

After a few days break from toning and strength work, your muscles are keen to get going again. There's an increase in the number of reps you'll be doing today. Don't be tempted to rush them – take a 30–45-second break between each exercise to recover properly.

1. Modified floor press ups: 1 set of 14 reps

2. Abdominal curls: 1 set of 14 reps

3. Half squats: 1 set of 14 reps

Stretch out your muscles afterwards to prevent tightening and soreness. Think about every stretch as you do it. Take time afterwards to relax and reflect on how well you're doing. Now that you've come this far, there's no going back!

FOOD FOR LIFE

Eating at home

If you hate cooking, fresh produce may just rot in your fridge. If you've got some cash to spend, you might prefer to buy ready meals from shops that specialise in healthy, whole foods. If you're on a tighter budget, perhaps you can set aside some time at weekends to prepare meals and freeze them to be reheated later that week. Why not visit your local bookshop or library? There are some excellent, healthy recipe books that focus on tasty meals that are cheap and easy to prepare.

If you're planning to eat good food at home, make sure you've got time to go shopping beforehand so you're not tempted to run out for fast food if the cupboards are bare.

Top shopping tips

◆ Set aside enough time to shop for a few days' worth of healthy food and ingredients.
◆ Make a list and stick to it.
◆ Don't go shopping when you're hungry.
◆ Once you're at the shop, stay away from the junk and the processed food aisles.
◆ Buy lots of fresh produce and choose lean meats and fish.
◆ Stay away from processed meats, fake cheese products and avoid the snack aisle.
◆ Shop for organic products whenever possible.
◆ If you can't shop regularly, choose frozen fruit and vegetables rather than canned foods, as they keep more of their nutrients.

TOP TIP 1

◆ Most people don't need to take vitamin supplements, because they get all the nutrients they need from a healthy, balanced diet. And popping pills can't give you the same benefits as eating well. Evidence suggests that fruit and vegetables are good for you not just because of the vitamins and minerals they contain, but because of the combination of different nutrients and fibre.

FOOD FOR LIFE

'Our own physical body possesses a wisdom which we who
inhabit the body lack. We give it orders which make no sense.'
Henry Miller, American writer

Activity

Active rest day

Be active and have fun. Don't worry about your
heart rate today!

- Take your dog for a long walk.

- Take the children or a loved on out for a
  leisurely stroll or bike ride.

- If it's cold outside, stay inside and put on your
  favourite CD or radio station. Do a little dance –
  a few twirls here... no one's looking!

- Wash the car... twice!

TOP TIP 2

- Exercise while running errands. When you go shopping,
  park towards the back of the car park and walk the extra
  distance. If you've got time, walk inside for a lap or two
  before you start shopping. Keep a pair of walking shoes
  in your car so that you're ready when you find any spare
  minutes for exercise.

MYTH: Your metabolism slows down once you hit
30.
FACT: Hundreds of research studies have shown
that a slow-down in metabolism is due to a loss of
muscle tissue. And the loss of muscle tissue is
directly related to a lack of hard physical activity.
So if you're 30+ but fit and active, your metabolism
will still be as quick as it always was!

FOOD FOR LIFE

Don't skip meals

Don't be too busy to look after yourself. If you skip breakfast, you may find that you wilt by mid-morning. Rather than missing breakfast completely, split it in half. Eat a small breakfast early, such as an egg, a small serving of oatmeal or some yoghurt. Then have a small snack on hand such as raisins and 10–12 almonds to eat mid-morning (have a look at the snack options in the weekly menu plans for more ideas). This is a much better solution than reaching for coffee or chocolate to perk you up.

TOP TIP 1

♦ Plan ahead. If you're going to a party straight after work, eat something before you go so that you don't dive into the nearest plate of snacks when you arrive. Go for something filling, such as a sandwich or a bowl of wholegrain cereal with skimmed or semi-skimmed milk.

MYTH: Pasta and bread are fattening.
FACT: Anything can be fattening! Lettuce can be stored as fat! Any food or drink that contains calories can be stored as body fat if it causes your blood-sugar levels to exceed what the body needs at that time. Bread and pasta are actually great sources of complex carbohydrate. The key is how much you eat and when you eat it.

FOOD FOR LIFE

Activity

Cardio 15-minute power walk

When out on your walk, try this easy and reliable test of exercise intensity. If you can easily chat with someone (or to yourself!) or sing along to music, you probably need to pick up the pace a little. But if you can't talk at all, you probably won't be able to keep this pace for long enough. For your walk to be aerobically challenging, you need to be somewhere in the middle of these two.

Now spend some quality time stretching and relaxing after your workout. Do all the stretches in Appendix 1 or choose your favourite ones, holding each one for as long as you wish.

TOP TIP 2

◆ Look good! If you feel good in your workout clothes, chances are you'll want to show them off! Buy yourself some outfits that make you feel good. No one said you had to workout in grimy T-shirts.

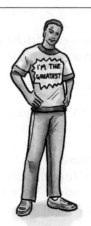

FOOD FOR LIFE

Control portion size

Our stomachs aren't really that big. Without being stretched, your stomach can hold about two cups of food, but because it *can* stretch, your tum can hold considerably more food at a meal than you need.

When you eat at home, serve your meals already dished up on plates rather than family style at the table. You'll be less likely to reach for seconds that way. At restaurants, ask for take-away containers and take half of your meal home. Avoid buffets, unless you're very disciplined. It's far too tempting to load up three or four plates plus pud!

Activity Active rest day

- Have you done the gardening yet? Give it a try.

- Use the stairs at least three times today.

- Leave something in your car that you'll need at some point during the day.

- Take the stairs to get from A to B.

- When you get home from work, do 100 marches on the spot before you sit and watch TV.

So exercise! The activity will tell your hypothalamus not to burn up your muscles (since you're using them) and to burn lots of calories by keeping your metabolism going fast.

'He who has health has hope and he who has hope has everything.' Thomas Carlyle, Scottish philosopher

TOP TIP 1

♦ No matter how busy your morning, don't forget breakfast. It only takes minutes to start your day with a delicious fruit shake. Blend 250ml (one cup) of fresh or frozen fruit with 125ml (half a cup) of low-fat yoghurt and 125 ml (half a cup) of fruit juice. Drink up and smile!

TOP TIP 2

♦ Schedule exercise as you would any other appointment. Don't change your exercise plans if something else comes along – remind yourself that exercise is just as important.

MYTH: When you're trying to lose weight, it's important to exercise.
FACT: True! It's very important to exercise. If you cut down on calories without exercising, your hypothalamus will think you're faced with a life-threatening shortage of food. It will slow down your metabolism, desperately trying to make your scarce resources (usually the protein in your muscles) last longer. Then you'll burn fewer calories in your sleep.

FOOD FOR LIFE

Tame your sweet tooth

Curb your cravings for sweets by eating fruit and staying away from sugary snacks and cakes. These treats have lots of calories, are loaded with unhealthy fats, plus some people seem to become addicted to these high-carb foods.

Your taste buds can learn to love fresh fruit without the added sweeteners. Avoid fizzy sweet drinks and try iced herbal teas or iced water with lemon or lime. If you miss the fizzy fix, add some fruit juice to sparkling water.

Activity

Cardio 16-minute power walk

Aim to do 16 minutes of walking today. Enjoy your time and the sensation of using and working your body – you can do it! Keep your back straight and walk tall. Look around you and relax into every stride – not too relaxed though! Changes and positive results take time and effort that only you can make. Don't forget to keep up a good challenging pace so that you benefit aerobically.

Don't skip the stretching, as you'll regret it. Very sore muscles after exercise indicate a lack of proper stretching – so go and find a tranquil place and do some stretches, paying particular attention to your legs.

'Happiness lies, first of all, in health.' George William Curtis, American social reformer, author and editor

TOP TIP 1

♦ Before you head out of the door every day always pack some fruit or veggie snacks in your bag or briefcase. Great portable options include apples, pears, bananas, clementines, baby carrots, cherry tomatoes, dried fruit and grapes.

TOP TIP 2

♦ If you have to travel to work, pack and plan so that you can keep up your exercise routine. Bring your skipping rope or choose a hotel that has fitness facilities. If you're stuck in an airport waiting for a plane, grab your hand luggage and take a walk.

MYTH: Performing aerobic exercise at low – rather than high – intensity promotes a greater loss of body fat.
FACT: It's true that the lower the intensity level at which you exercise, the more the body prefers to use fats rather than carbohydrates as fuel. But the *total amount* of fat calories burned during high-intensity exercise tends to be equal to or greater than the number burned during low-intensity exercise, even though the *percentage* of calories burned from fat is higher during low-intensity exercise.

FOOD FOR LIFE

Things you don't want to give up

Do you feel like you can't live without your chocolate… that or your mornings just can't begin without a cup of coffee? If there are foods you don't want to give up, enjoy them in smaller amounts. For example, buy one tiny, high-quality piece of choccie and enjoy it, but don't buy a bag full of snacks to take with you. Switch to decaffeinated coffee or at least drink an extra glass of water for every cup of coffee you have. The caffeine is a diuretic, which means it makes your body lose water. With other treats or favourite foods that aren't healthy, try to limit them to once a week or search for healthier versions at health food shops.

Activity

Mobility exercises/ toning and strength

You're getting stronger and shapelier now. The workouts are paying dividends. You no longer look as if you're about to take off if you flap your arms! Can you see and feel the tone in your arms? As for your legs – bye, bye thunder thighs. Haven't you noticed that bag for a belly is no more? Stick with this toning work and your shape will change forever. Today, to get your legs in even greater shape, you'll change your squats exercise for an even more effective form. Make sure you warm up first, and then give them a go!

1. Modified floor press ups: 1 set of 14 reps

2. Abdominal curls: 1 set of 14 reps

3. Chair leg squats: 1 set of 10 reps

Now give your body the stretching it deserves after a good blitzing!

'Body: a thing of shreds and patches, borrowed unequally from good and bad ancestors and a misfit from the start.'
Ralph Waldo Emerson, American author, poet and philosopher

TOP TIP 1

♦ Buy convenience food at the supermarket. Never before have there been so many pre-peeled, pre-cut and ready-to-eat goodies available. Stock up on washed and bagged salads, baby carrots, celery hearts, broccoli and cauliflower crowns, cherry tomatoes, shredded cabbage, salad-bar delights, sliced mushrooms, roasted red peppers (in a jar) and ready-made dips for veggies or fruit. Eating more vegetables has never been so easy!

TOP TIP 2

♦ Make your exercise routine work for your lifestyle. One challenge is finding and making the time to do it. Try watching TV while using a treadmill, or read a magazine or book while pedalling on a stationary bike.

MYTH: You can burn fat from specific areas of the body by exercising those areas.
FACT: Contrary to what you may want to believe, the phenomenon of 'spot reduction' has absolutely no factual basis. When you exercise, you utilise energy produced by metabolising fat from *all* of the regions of your body – not just the specific muscles involved in exercise.

FOOD FOR LIFE

Rome wasn't built in a day

If you can't transform your unhealthy diet overnight, don't despair. Most people can't. Start implementing some of these ideas, even just one at a time. Every change you make will be one step in the right direction.

Activity

Cardio 17-minute power walk

You'll feel much better from the hard effort you've put in and the changes you've made in your lifestyle. Remember, you're doing this for all the right reasons. Today, get used to walking slightly faster, holding yourself more upright than you usually do – this extra pace makes all the difference. It may be a bit difficult, but hang in there. Regulate your breathing and make sure you lead with your heel and roll through to the ball of your foot. Go for it!

Don't miss out your stretches otherwise you'll only end up feeling stiff and sore tomorrow. While stretching, reflect on how well you've done and how far you can go. Use this time for positive thoughts as you move from one stretch to the next.

TOP TIP 1

◆ Set performance goals. People who can stick with a new behaviour for six months usually make it a habit.

'I am convinced digestion is the great secret to life.' Sydney Smith, English clergyman and essayist

 TOP TIP 2

♦ Use your microwave. It's fast. It's easy. It's one of the best ways to preserve nutrients when cooking vegetables. And remember – for perfect veggies, remove them from the microwave when they're barely tender and let them stand for three to five minutes to finish cooking.

MYTH: Some people are too old to workout.
FACT: You're never too old – you can start exercising at any age. Recent strength-training studies show that people in their 80s can benefit from exercise.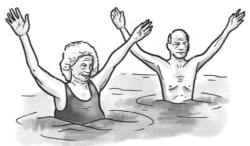
But do check with your doctor before starting an exercise programme, especially if you're over 45. If you've never exercised before or have a health condition such as diabetes or heart disease, think about working with a qualified personal trainer to get you started. The trainer should have experience in training people who are your age and at your level of fitness.

FOOD FOR LIFE

Your notes

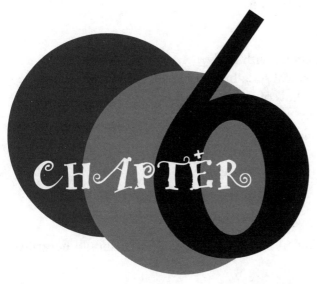

CHAPTER 6

CULINARY
CONCOCTIONS

You can speed up the weight-loss process simply by sticking with your eating plan. How have you done so far? Surely a size smaller! For even better results keep up the good work in Week 4.

Breakfast

Choose one of the following breakfast suggestions every day. Each option contains 280–300 calories.

◆ Medium bowl of cereal with milk
  One slice of wholemeal soda bread or toast with jam/marmalade
  One small glass (100ml) of unsweetened or fresh fruit juice (100ml)
  Choose this option for at least four days this week.
◆ Two slices of apple, raisin and sultana loaf lightly covered with olive-oil spread
  One small glass (100ml) of orange juice
◆ Porridge/toasted oat cereal
  Fresh fruit
  Tea
◆ Traditional breakfast (if it's a cooked breakfast, it should be grilled rather than fried)

Mid-morning/mid-afternoon snack

Choose one of the following snacks each day. It doesn't matter whether you have it at 10am, 3pm or 10pm but it makes sense to choose a time when you think you'll enjoy it most. For example, if you start work at 8am and don't have lunch until 1pm, mid-morning is probably the best time to have your snack. If you normally work late and don't have dinner until late evening, a mid-afternoon snack will keep you going.

Each snack contains 60–100 calories.

- One digestive biscuit
- Two crackers
- One small bowl of fresh fruit salad
- One small slice of fruit cake
- Two fig rolls
- Diet fruit yoghurt

Lunch/light meal

If it suits you to eat your main meal at lunch time or if, for example, you're going out to a restaurant for lunch, skip forward to the main meal section for suggestions. It doesn't make any difference to your diet whether you eat your main meal in the evening or at lunch time. But, it's important to eat something at lunch time to prevent snacking on high-calorie foods later on in the day.

The options listed below each contain 400–450 calories.

Sandwiches

Enjoy a sandwich for lunch for six days this week. Choose your filling from these options:

- Low-fat cheddar cheese with relish on wholemeal/granary bread (two slices bread and 30g grated cheese)
  Fresh fruit
  Tea/mineral water/fruit juice
- ★Smoked salmon open sandwich on wholemeal soda bread (two slices) with a green salad and lemon wedge
  Fresh fruit
  Tea/mineral water/fruit juice
- ★Chicken, sweetcorn and lettuce on wholegrain sliced bread (two slices)
  Fresh fruit
  Tea/mineral water/fruit juice

CULINARY CONCOCTIONS

- Spiced beef and horseradish sauce open sandwich made with two slices of wholemeal soda bread, two wafer-thin slices of beef and one teaspoonful of horseradish sauce
Fresh fruit
Tea/mineral water/fruit juice
- Three slices of turkey breast with iceberg lettuce on ciabatta bread
Fresh fruit
Tea/mineral water/fruit juice

★ Choose either low-fat mayonnaise or olive-oil spread on your bread for these sandwiches, but not both. For all other sandwich suggestions, avoid salad dressing and butter.

Other lunch option

- Large bowl of low-fat vegetable soup
Ham sandwich with two slices of wholemeal bread
Fresh fruit
Tea/cappuccino (made with skimmed milk)

Tip

Grated cheese goes much further when making sandwiches.

Main meal

You can choose to eat this meal earlier in the day and have a light meal from the lunch menu later – it's up to you.

These main meal suggestions contain 450–600 calories.

- *Pasta and salad*
Pasta with tomato-based sauce (ready-to-serve sauce) and large green salad.

Allow five handfuls of dried uncooked pasta per portion and enjoy one dessert spoonful of flavoured salad dressing oil on the salad. Avoid cream and oil-based pasta sauces!

◆ *Spaghetti bolognaise*
Use three dessert spoonfuls of bolognaise, made from good-quality mince, per portion. Don't add any oil to the mince when frying. Serve with lots of spaghetti. Make up extra bolognaise sauce so that you can freeze it and use as a topping on baked potatoes on another day.

◆ *Two large baked potatoes*
Serve with bolognaise or chilli topping and side salad. Dry roast the potatoes on the top shelf of the oven on a lightly salted tray.

◆ *Fish pie*
Allow 110–140g cooked weight of fish per portion. Lightly steam the fish first. Transfer to an ovenproof dish and top with mashed potatoes (mash potatoes with milk only) Bake in the oven until golden brown. Serve with a small portion of tinned beans or peas.

◆ *Stir-fry chicken*
Stir-fry six cubes of a chicken portion in olive oil and add onions and carrots. Add three dessert spoonfuls of ready made sweet chilli sauce and bean sprouts at the end of cooking. Serve with rice and a side salad.

◆ *Omelette*
Make with two or three eggs and fry with a knob of low-fat butter. Fill with onion, tomato and 15 grams of grated low-fat cheddar. Serve with a side salad.

Note – side salad

Use a combination of all or some of the following: lettuce (all types), rocket, scallions, cucumber, peppers, tomatoes, but no dressing unless stated.

CULINARY CONCOCTIONS

'I am dying with the help of too many physicians.'
Alexander the Great

Get an oil change

While all cooking oils are 100% fat and contain about 40 calories a teaspoonful, some are better than others. One reason why the rate of heart disease is lower in countries like Greece and Italy is because monounsaturated, fat-rich olive oil is a staple in the Mediterranean diet.

Types of fats

Monounsaturated fats – 'monos'

- Help lower LDL cholesterol levels, without lowering high-density lipoprotein (HDL), the so-called 'good' cholesterol.
- Less likely to be oxidised than 'polys' – oxidised fatty acids of LDLs deposit LDL into the walls of arteries.

Found in fish oil, nuts olive oil and flaxseed oil.

Polyunsaturated fats – 'polys'

- Help lower LDL cholesterol levels, but also lower high-density lipoprotein (HDL), the so-called 'good' cholesterol.
- More likely to be oxidised.

Traditional fats – butter, lard and vegetable shortening – are all high in dangerous saturated or trans fats. The worst oils are the so-called 'tropical' oils like coconut and palm oil. Unfortunately, they're used a lot in processed and snack foods because they add texture and flavour to foods.

Activity

Active rest day

Try these activities to be more active and have a little fun:

● Yoga

● Pilates

● Belly dancing

● Ballroom dancing

● Walk, run, play... or just move around more than usual!

TOP TIP

◆ Remember – a calorie is a calorie. High-fat foods generally have more calories than foods that are high in carbohydrates or protein, but the best way to lose weight is to eat fewer calories than you burn every day. While you can eat larger quantities of foods that are low in fat – as long as they're also low in calories – do check labels or read nutritional guidance in magazines or from the internet to make sure they're good for you.

MYTH: Protein builds muscle.
FACT: Exercise builds muscle. Protein is used to help repair the damage to the muscle from exercise or over exertion.

CULINARY CONCOCTIONS

Eat fewer animal foods

Animal foods like meat (unless it's very lean) and dairy products tend to be rich in saturated fats. They're also high in cholesterol, which is only found in animal foods, not plant foods. Eat no more than three servings of meat a week and choose the leanest cuts such as beef fillet, loin, sirloin, pork loin chops, turkey and chicken. All cuts with the name 'loin' or 'fillet' are lean. And if you cook it yourself, trim all visible fat and drain the grease.

Focus your dairy intake on yoghurt products rather than butter or cream.

TOP TIP 1

♦ Whenever you put food in your mouth, peel it, unwrap it, put it on a plate and sit down and enjoy it! Use all your senses to relish the fact that what you're eating is nourishing your body.

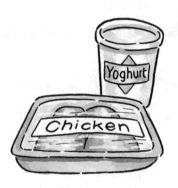

'Leading a sedentary and unhealthy lifestyle is asking for trouble – before you know it, your body will start to call it a day.'
Cornel Chin

CULINARY CONCOCTIONS

Activity

Cardio 18-minute walk

Feeling good now I bet! Think about how the walk makes you feel and get really plugged into the exercise. You should feel full of energy and stimulated afterwards, so make it a good one. Walk tall, keeping your ribcage lifted and stomach muscles pulled in. Don't forget to breathe normally throughout.

When you've finished your walk, spend some time stretching out all of your muscles.

TOP TIP 2

♦ Think positively. Don't let negative self-talk, such as 'I'm a failure' get in the way of starting again if you have to skip a workout or two. Shrug it off as a temporary break in your walking programme.

MYTH: Some fancy new exercise machine burns more calories than any other exercise.
FACT: Many people seem confused about how many calories are burnt during different types of exercise. Don't be fooled into thinking a new machine can burn more calories. The bottom line is that how many calories you burn is directly related to the amount of effort you put into an activity. In general, the more difficult it feels, the more calories you burn. The easier it feels the fewer calories you burn. Simple. So get working hard!

CULINARY CONCOCTIONS

Read food labels

By reading food labels, you'll be able to see which products contain harmful oils. And you'll see exactly how much more fat and how many more calories you're eating. Many canned and packaged products may seem like a single serving, but can contain two or more recommended servings. And since labelled fat and calorie content is calculated on the recommended portion size, you may be eating two or three times as much fat and calories as you think!

Avoid saturated fats

Reading labels for terms like 'hydrogenated' can also make you aware of trans fats. Hydrogenation adds hydrogen to an unsaturated (and less harmful) fat to give a product more texture. Hydrogenation turns a vegetable oil, which most people consider safer, into one that can raise cholesterol as much as animal fats. So keep an eye out for the words 'hydrogenated' or 'partially hydrogenated' on packets of biscuits, cakes and snacks, as well as sweets and other products.

Reading labels also helps you calculate your total fat calories and, perhaps even more importantly, your intake of saturated fats, which should comprise no more than 10% of your total calories. So if you're consuming 2,000 calories a day, you should have no more than 22 grams of saturated fat.

TOP TIP 1

♦ Eat when you're hungry and stop when you're full. Eat smaller portions. Never help yourself to seconds.

TOP TIP 2

♦ Women need fewer calories than men because women have more body fat than men and fat metabolises more slowly than lean body mass. A cast-iron way for women to speed up their metabolism is to exercise more!

CULINARY CONCOCTIONS

90

Activity

Mobility exercises/ toning and strength

It's good for your tone, it's good for your muscles and it's good for your bones! It can sometimes feel like a tall order, but results come from effort, time and commitment. Remember those words from a famous advert, 'Because you're worth it!'

When performing these toners today, focus on strict technique. Feel and think about your muscles really working. Channel your energy into each and every rep. Watch out for the change in reps today!

1. Modified floor press ups: 1 set of 15 reps

2. Abdominal curls: 1 set of 15 reps

3. Chair leg squats: 1 set of 15 reps

Challenging exercises result in challenged muscles, so give them a chance to recover by finishing off with a set of stretching.

MYTH: Aerobic exercise tends to make you hungry, so it actually undermines your efforts to lose weight. **FACT:** Aerobic exercise, such as jogging or brisk walking, may increase your appetite – but only, it seems, if you need extra calories. Studies suggest that lean individuals do get hungrier after such exercise – it stops them getting too thin. By contrast, working out doesn't seem to boost appetite in overweight individuals – so exercise should help them slim down.

CULINARY CONCOCTIONS

Are you keeping up? Do you need some help? If you've not already subscribed, why not try the daily text messaging service for extra encouragement and support.
Just text 'Body Idol 31' to 80881 now.

Each set of messages costs £1.50. Please see page xiv for full terms and conditions.

Fat substitutes

Fat substitutes give reduced-fat and fat-free versions of foods a flavour, texture and appearance similar to that of the original food. Although they may not suit all palettes, these substitutes are certainly a healthier alternative. Some fat substitutes are carbohydrate-based and others are protein-based. They're used individually or in combination in all kinds of foods, including margarine, salad dressings, cheese and other dairy products, and frozen desserts. Food manufacturers use fat substitutes to make foods that are not only lower in total fat, but also in saturated fat, cholesterol and calories. Both carbohydrate-based and protein-based substitutes contribute calories, but usually fewer than those contained in fat.

The carbohydrate-based fat substitutes you might see listed on a food label include modified starches, dextrin, cellulose and gums. When combined with water, these products swell and can be used to thicken foods, such as fat-free mayonnaise and salad dressings. Protein-based fat substitutes are made from skimmed-milk protein. They lend a creamy texture to foods such as low-fat ice cream and frozen yoghurt. Milk protein is also used to improve the texture and appearance of reduced-fat cheeses.

> **MYTH:** All fat is bad.
> **FACT:** Our bodies need fat for vital functioning. It helps slow the ageing process and satisfies hunger for long periods of time – up to five hours. The key is to replace the unhealthy fats in your diet with healthy fats such as olive oil.

CULINARY CONCOCTIONS

'A person always has two reasons for doing anything: a good reason and the real reason.' John Pierpont Morgan, American banker and financier

Activity

Cardio 19-minute power walk

You're really progressing well now, but don't rest on your laurels. Keep the pace up so you feel slightly breathless – this encourages your body to use more energy and burn fat. Pump with those arms as you take long strides with your legs, landing on your heels first and following through onto the balls of your feet.

Afterwards, stretch those eager muscles. Why not hold each stretch for a little longer? This will increase muscle tone and flexibility, and will also help you to let go of any strains and stresses from the day.

TOP TIP 1

♦ Choose wisely. If you haven't got time to eat before a party, chose your snacks carefully. Breadsticks are a great choice but watch out for those dips. An average portion of houmous contains 6g of fat and 90 calories. The same amount of taramasalata has 25g of fat and 250 calories.

TOP TIP 2

♦ Don't get intimidated by the prospect of a daily exercise regime. You don't have to run a marathon. You need only get your body moving every day. Once you tone your muscles, you'll naturally find yourself wanting to do more challenging workouts.

CULINARY CONCOCTIONS

Stick to non-stick pans

Cooking oils bump up your fat intake and calories, so why not try using non-stick pans rather than oil? Or try a little orange juice to prevent food from sticking. Instead of oil or butter, use small amounts of water, wine or stock to sauté food, and adapt recipes to use cooking methods that naturally reduce fat, such as boiling or simmering, grilling, roasting, poaching, microwaving, steaming or stir-frying.

Activity

Active rest day

Today is a rest day, although do a workout if you really must! A rest day means active rest so you still need to move around throughout the day. Try walking a little more, and stretching while you're watching TV or doing something fun with your family and friends. You could give a yoga video or DVD a go for a relaxing workout. You know the drill... move more, play more and sit less!

TOP TIP 1

- ♦ If you love dips and can't bear to eat breadsticks naked, why not make your own low-fat dips? A tasty one to try is a chilli bean dip. Mix up half a tin of red kidney beans with a raw onion, a garlic clove and a red chilli; add a dash of lemon juice and a pinch each of cumin, dry mustard and salt. A good-sized portion contains just 0.5g of fat.

CULINARY CONCOCTIONS

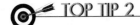

TOP TIP 2

♦ Make sure you're doing it right. One reason for wanting to give up exercise is injury or pain. Check with your doctor if you feel any pain. And check in with fitness trainers, too, if you're working on equipment at the gym or trying a new sport.

MYTH: Crash diets work.
FACT: No crash diet works. Anyone can go on a very low-calorie diet and lose five kilos quickly. There are plenty of diets designed for initial weight loss, usually eating less than 1,000 calories a day. But studies show that people who diet in this way usually put it all back on within a year. More importantly, vital nutrients are lacking in a very low-calorie diet. The moment you cut down on calories, your body is given signals that it's starving and slows down, burning fewer calories. To your slowed-down body those 800 calories will feel like 8,000, so you can actually start regaining weight on 800 to 1,000 calories a day! When you start eating your usual amount again, your body will have slowed down so much it won't be able to speed up in time to bump off the extra food you eat. So the food goes right into your fat cells – usually on your buttocks, thighs and stomach.

CULINARY CONCOCTIONS

Sensible foods

Below is an overview of healthy foods. Photocopy this page and stick it on your fridge or cupboard door.

Poor eating

◆ Battered and deep-fried foods
◆ Sugary treats
◆ Processed meats
◆ Greasy snacks
◆ White bread and pasta

Good eating

◆ Green and brightly coloured vegetables
◆ Fresh fruit
◆ Lean meats and fish
◆ Nuts, raisins and healthy snacks
◆ Wholegrain breads and pasta

Great eating!

◆ Raw or lightly steamed vegetables with no heavy sauces
◆ Organic fruit and vegetables
◆ Organic lean meat and poultry
◆ Oily ocean fish

'It is a mistake to look too far ahead. Only one link in the
chain of destiny can be handled at a time.'
Sir Winston Churchill, British orator, author and Prime Minister

CULINARY CONCOCTIONS

Activity

Cardio 20-minute power walk

20 minutes of walking should fit quite comfortably into your daily schedule now. Keep walking at a pace that encourages you to breathe slightly more heavily, while increasing your body temperature at the same time. Take in the fresh air and energise yourself!

During your stretching, reflect on your successes and achievements so far. Apply some creative visualisation – think only constructive thoughts as you breathe in and breathe out any negative thoughts.

TOP TIP

◆ If you're having a low-energy day, only exercise for 10 minutes. That will get you moving and, once you're in the groove, you'll usually want to finish your workout.

MYTH: Writing things down doesn't make any difference in helping to achieve goals.
FACT: It does! People who are committed to keeping track of what they eat and drink – and their daily activity – succeed. It's so easy to pop something into your mouth and then say, 'It was small, it doesn't count.' But, if you write things down, you can clearly see where your biggest weak spots are. You can then start taking steps to change them, one at a time. And that's the secret to long-term success – baby steps!

CULINARY CONCOCTIONS

Reality check

A clear weight-loss goal

It's natural to want a clear weight-loss goal. Some ways of assessing your weight include BMI (body-mass index), waist-to-hip ratio and weighing yourself (all covered in detail in Appendix 2). Goal weights should vary from person to person according to your gender, body frame and height.

But remember, you can't control some factors affecting your weight – the chief one being genetics. Research has shown that hereditary factors may increase your weight by up to 30%. Other 'uncontrollable' issues include weight gain due to side effects from medication, extreme inactivity due to medical problems and thyroid/metabolic conditions.

Percentage of body fat

Your percentage of body fat is another important measure. A doctor or exercise professional can work this out. Using an instrument called a calliper, they measure the thickness of a fold of skin (for example, on the back of the arm) to estimate your total body fat. The average European woman of normal weight has 20–30% body fat. Trained athletes usually have less while pregnant women tend to have more.

Exercise more!

Although there are many programmes to help you lose weight, the only proven long-term and safe method is to burn more calories than you consume. You can achieve this either by reducing your calorie intake (eating less or healthier food) or by increasing you energy expenditure (exercising more). Once you've lost weight, you can modify your habits slightly to keep the weight off.

Activity

Mobility exercises/toning and strength

Today two exercises have been replaced with newer, more intense toners. An extra exercise has been added to target the 'bingo wings' (backs of the arms) that can sometimes be hard to change. Your reps vary for each exercise, so don't get too carried away. Try more if you're finding them easy. Here goes!

1. Floor arm dips: 1 set of 10 reps

2. Modified floor press ups: 1 set of 12 reps

3. Curls ups: 1 set of 15 reps

4. Chair leg squats: 1 set of 15 reps

Don't forget to stretch afterwards and pay special attention to the arms, otherwise you'll feel it tomorrow.

TOP TIP 1

♦ If time is short, spend an extra bit of cash to buy vegetables that are already washed and cut up.

TOP TIP 2

♦ Use a visible reward system. The effects of exercise are cumulative and long term, so sometimes it helps to see your results on a daily basis. After every workout, put a big red star on your calendar or in your diary as a symbol that you've completed the day's workout. Take photos of yourself every month in your workout gear so you've also got a visual record of your results.

CULINARY CONCOCTIONS

Your notes

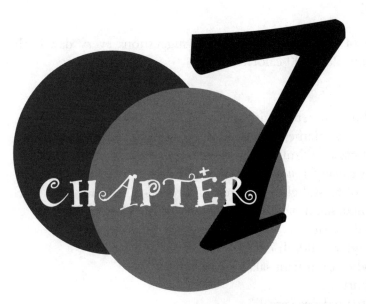

CHAPTER 7

COMBATING STRESS AND CALORIES!

This is the final stage of your healthy eating plan. You now hold the keys to successful eating and know how to prepare delicious and healthy food quickly and easily. You'll now bring your 'kick start' programme to an end with Week 5 – but don't forget to keep up the good work by producing your own menu plans.

Breakfast

Choose one of the following breakfast suggestions every day. Each option contains 280–300 calories.

♦ Medium bowl of cereal with milk
  One slice of wholemeal soda bread or toast with jam/marmalade
  One small glass (100ml) of unsweetened or fresh fruit juice
  Choose this option for at least four days this week.
♦ Two slices of toast, lightly covered with olive-oil spread
  One poached/scrambled egg
  One grilled tomato
  One small glass (100ml) of orange juice
  Large bowl of fresh fruit salad
  Fruit yoghurt
♦ Porridge/toasted oat cereal
  Fresh fruit
  Tea/herbal tea

Mid-morning/mid-afternoon snack

Choose one of the following snacks each day. It doesn't matter whether you have it at 10am, 3pm or 10pm but it makes sense to choose a time when you think you'll enjoy it most. For example, if you start work at 8am and don't have lunch until 1pm, mid-morning is probably the best time to have your snack. If you normally work late and don't have dinner until late evening, a mid-afternoon snack will keep you going.

Each snack contains 60–100 calories.

- One apple
- Two chocolate chip cookies
- One small bowl of fresh fruit salad
- Two satsumas
- One digestive biscuit
- Diet fruit yoghurt

Lunch/light meal

If it suits you to eat your main meal at lunch time or if, for example, you're going out to a restaurant for lunch, skip forward to the main meal section for suggestions. It doesn't make any difference to your diet whether you eat your main meal in the evening or at lunch time. But, it's important to eat something at lunch time to prevent snacking on high-calorie foods later on in the day.

The options listed below each contain 400–450 calories.

Sandwiches

Enjoy a sandwich for lunch for six days of this week. Choose your filling from these options.

- Turkey curry wrap with lettuce and peppers using two slices of turkey, 10g (two teaspoonfuls) low-fat curry mayonnaise, iceberg lettuce, peppers, one flour tortilla
  Fruit
  Fruit juice/mineral water
- Brie cheese and chutney sandwich with two slices of wholemeal soda bread, using small triangle of brie, three teaspoonfuls (15g) chutney
  Fruit
  Fruit juice/mineral water

- Roasted peppers with salsa and sour cream in a wrap, using roasted peppers, three dessert spoonfuls of salsa (homemade if possible), 10g (two teaspoonfuls) sour cream/crème fraiche or natural bio yoghurt, one flour tortilla
  Fresh fruit
  Cappuccino (made with skimmed milk)/flavoured mineral water/tea/fruit juice
- *Tuna, sweetcorn and lettuce on wholegrain sliced bread (two slices)
  Fresh fruit
  Tea/mineral water/fruit juice
- Spiced beef and horseradish sauce, open sandwich made with two slices of wholemeal soda bread, two wafer-thin slices of beef and one teaspoonful of horseradish sauce
  Fresh fruit
  Tea/mineral water/fruit juice
- *Three slices of honey-roast ham with iceberg lettuce on white batch bread
  Fresh fruit
  Tea/mineral water/fruit juice

* Choose either low-fat mayonnaise or olive-oil spread on your bread for these sandwiches, but not both. For all other sandwich suggestions, neither salad dressing nor butter is recommended.

Tip

Grated cheese goes much further when making up sandwiches.

Main meal

You can choose to eat this meal earlier in the day and have a light meal from the lunch menu later – it's up to you.

The main meal suggestions below contain 450–600 calories.

- *Turkey fajitas*
  Use two flour tortillas per portion, filled with diced turkey, onion, lettuce, peppers, chilli and garlic. Add a tin of tomatoes when cooking the onion, peppers, chilli and garlic. Toss in the diced cooked turkey to heat through when all the other ingredients are cooked.

- *Pasta and ratatouille*
  Allow five handfuls of dried uncooked pasta shapes per portion. Add a large portion of ratatouille (homemade if possible) to the cooked pasta and serve with 30g of low-fat cheddar cheese grated on top.

- *Stew*
  Irish stew/beef casserole with two medium-sized boiled potatoes.

- *Burger and chips*
  Homemade 100g beef burger and oven chips. Use good-quality mince for the burger. Add seasoning and half a chopped onion. Fry in olive oil and serve in a toasted bun with 100g (cooked weight) of oven chips (small portion). Enjoy with a side salad.

- *Stir-fry chicken*
  Stir-fry six cubes of a chicken portion in one calorie spray oil and add onions and carrots. Add three dessert spoonfuls of readymade sauce and bean sprouts at the end of cooking. Serve with rice and a side salad.

- *Omelette*
  Made with two or three eggs fried in a knob of low-fat butter and filled with onion, tomato, onion and diced ham. Serve with a side salad.

- *Roast dinner*
  Roast dinner of beef, lamb or pork. Turkey and chicken have featured widely this week so go for a roasted meat dish. Have two large slices of meat with two boiled potatoes and two fresh or frozen vegetables. Make gravy from granules or stock, not meat juice, as this contains a lot of fat.

COMBATING STRESS AND CALORIES!

Get a grip and overcome stress

Stress is a normal part of life. You need to be stressed to some extent to perform any task. When we feel stress, adrenal glands secrete various hormones that are important in helping the body function. Cortisol, one of these hormones, controls various stress reactions. You need to know how to control demands in your life, without letting them get out of the control. When this happens, the adrenal glands release too many hormones, and end up getting worn out.

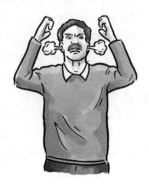

Common causes of stress

♦ Moving home
♦ Bereavement
♦ A relationship break-up or divorce
♦ Changing jobs
♦ Juggling family and work commitments
♦ A fear of failure
♦ Demanding children.

TOP TIP

♦ Sports count too. If you hate the thought of going out to exercise today, find something you do like. Start a badminton or netball league at work. Learn to play tennis. You'll have fun and, guess what? You'll be exercising!

'Let nothing which can be treated by diet be treated by other means.' Maimonides, Jewish rabbi, physician and philosopher

Activity

Cardio 21-minute power walk

You're about to achieve a major milestone today – a 21-minute walk is a big breakthrough. You should be very proud that you've stuck with this programme, but you can head for even greater heights! Now as you power through your walk today, keep your back straight and be aware of how tall you're walking. Relax your face and try smiling – be happy in the knowledge that a new you is beginning to emerge!

When you've finished, ease out of your workout by doing stretches that focus on your legs, chest and stomach.

MYTH: Carbohydrates (or sugars) cause weight gain.
FACT: Carbohydrates don't cause weight gain unless they contribute to excess calorie intake. The same holds true for protein and fat. People who successfully lose weight tend to eat diets that are higher in carbohydrates and lower in fat, as well as watching their total calorie intake. But some people who eat a diet that's extremely high in carbohydrates and low in protein and fat get hungry sooner, which may trigger overeating.

COMBATING STRESS AND CALORIES!

Test your stress

Today, complete the Life Stress test from Appendix 3. Make sure you treat the results as a useful guide rather than as a precise survey. Complete it quickly and don't think too hard before answering each question. Your first response is often the most accurate one. It isn't difficult to spot what the 'low stress' answers are so don't be tempted to give them if they're not the right ones! The purpose of the test is simply to help you clarify some of your thinking about your own life. Finally, a test you *don't* want a high score on!

Activity
Active rest day

Have you bought a pedometer? If not, hit your local department store or sports shop and pick one up. They're inexpensive and really useful. Keep track of how many steps you're walking and try to increase the number every day.

'The doctor of the future will give no medication, but will interest his patients in the care of the human frame, diet and in the cause and prevention of disease.' Thomas Edison, scientist and inventor

TOP TIP 1

♦ Don't go to a party or event on an empty stomach. Skipping meals means you're hungry and your chances of overeating later are much higher. Before going out, snack on protein, like chicken or cottage cheese. Protein satisfies and helps you eat less.

COMBATING STRESS AND CALORIES!

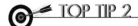

TOP TIP 2

◆ Reward! Reward! Reward! If you find exercise is torture, give yourself something for getting through it. Whether you exercise for four days in a row or jog an extra mile – if you're happy with your performance, give yourself a prize. This could be a day off from exercise, a new pair of jeans... make yourself happy because you deserve it!

MYTH: The more you sweat during exercise, the more fat you lose.

FACT: The harder you workout, the more calories you'll burn and so the more fat you stand to lose. But how much you sweat doesn't necessarily reflect how hard you're working. Some people tend to sweat a lot due to heavy body weight, poor conditioning or hereditary factors. And everyone sweats more in hot, dry weather or dense clothing than in cool, humid weather or porous clothing. (You may feel as if you're sweating more in humid weather; but that's because moist air slows the evaporation of sweat.) Exercising in extremely hot weather or in a plastic 'weight loss' suit will make you sweat heavily and lose weight immediately. But that lost weight is almost entirely water – the kilos will return when you replenish your fluids by drinking after the workout. You're also in danger of getting heat exhaustion if you push yourself too hard in extreme heat or in plastic clothes, which prevent sweat from evaporating and stop you cooling off.

COMBATING STRESS AND CALORIES!

How to cope with stress

Exercise regularly

Plan your leisure time for maximum health and enjoyment. Your body needs daily exercise. This is particularly true of those who have a sedentary lifestyle.

Talk positively to yourself

Talk to yourself (when you're alone!), giving yourself positive and encouraging feedback when you do the right thing. Every day try things like:

'I'm really pleased with how I did this morning.'
'I handled that issue with X pretty well just now.'
'That was a great workout session, well done!'

Statements like this can go a long way in building your self-esteem and you get a more realistic view of yourself. Once you gain a strong feeling of self-worth, your ability to handle stress rises considerably.

Eat wisely

You are what you eat. Aim for nourishing, regular meals, made up mostly of vegetables, fruits and cereals, with moderate amounts of lean meat, dairy, nuts and eggs. You can also include a small amount of butter, margarine, and oil but avoid sugar and salt. Drink plenty of water – at least eight glasses a day in hot weather. Avoid coffee, tea and soft drinks as much as possible. And remember not to skip breakfast!

Support network

A problem shared is a problem solved. Use your personal support network, such as friends, family or work colleagues, to talk through any problems or concerns.

Sleep and relaxation exercises

Lack of sleep can lead to extra stress and this can lead to depression. Combat it with a good night's sleep most nights. There will be the occasional night when you're up late, but always balance it with late mornings or early nights.

COMBATING STRESS AND CALORIES!

Systematic relaxation exercises as well as controlled deep breathing have been shown to help composure, reduce anxiety and refresh most people. Since reaction to stress and strain is muscle tension, the obvious remedy is occasional but deliberate muscle relaxation.

Activity

Cardio 22-minute power walk

Keep your walk energetic, and challenge your body to walk faster. If you come to a slight hill, make the effort to feel your buttocks working too and pump those arms to help you get up there. Keep your posture upright and stomach muscles taught. Lift your chest high and take in huge lungfuls of air. Stoke up the fuel burners and get those muscles working!

After a good high-energy workout, you'll look forward to giving your body the stretches it deserves and to spend some quiet time relaxing into every stretch.

TOP TIP 1

◆ Don't skip meals. Many healthy eaters with good intentions diet by day and binge by night. You're only fooling yourself.

TOP TIP 2

◆ Read health and fitness books or magazines to inspire you. Feel motivated by the stories and profiles of those who have succeeded in their health and fitness goals.

COMBATING STRESS AND CALORIES!

Calories and reality

Are you unhappy with your weight? Have you ever looked in the mirror and asked, 'How did I get to be this size?' Well, the explanation is deceptively simple: if you consume more calories than you need on a daily basis, the excess calories turn into extra weight. Think of food as fuel and your body as a car. Food is the energy our bodies run on. Overeating is like over-fuelling and the excess fuel turns into fat. In this way, the cycle of weight gain starts.

The core principle of weight loss is just as straightforward as that of weight gain. If you eat fewer calories than you burn, you'll lose weight. This is the basis of every weight-loss diet. Whether you follow a low-fat or low-carbohydrate/high protein diet, or you reduce portion sizes, these are all means to the same end: fewer calories consumed. Over the next few days, you'll have the opportunity to increase your knowledge and discover some useful facts about calories.

'The belly is ungrateful – it always forgets we already gave it something.' Russian proverb

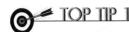 TOP TIP 1

♦ Brush your teeth straight after dinner to remind yourself that you've finished eating for the night. And brush after every meal too!

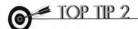 TOP TIP 2

♦ Re-evaluate your goals. If your goal is to walk two hours a day for 365 days a year, you might be setting yourself up to fail. Set realistic goals for yourself, such as 30 minutes of exercise, five days a week.

COMBATING STRESS AND CALORIES!

Activity

Mobility exercises/toning and strength

You've got to do more today so make a conscious effort to focus your mind on the muscles you're working. Keep following the descriptions and studying the illustrations in Appendix 2 until you feel confident that you're working the right muscles and that your posture and technique are correct and supportive.

1. Floor arm dips: 1 set of 12 reps

2. Modified floor press ups: 1 set of 14 reps

3. Curls ups: 1 set of 16 reps

4. Chair leg squats: 1 set of 16 reps

Your muscles will be tired from your efforts so they deserve a good relaxing stretch.

MYTH: Yoghurt is the perfect diet food.
FACT: Yoghurt is, indeed, important for those wanting to lose weight. It's naturally rich in calcium, which research has shown helps to reduce weight gain. Even small changes in the calcium levels of fat cells can change signals within the cells that control the making and burning of fat. Avoid yoghurt with added sugars or sweetened fruit, as these upset the delicate chemical balance that allows the cultures to thrive. Sugar also feeds the growth of unwanted yeasts, so you're better off without it! Avoid Greek yoghurt too, which has 10% fat.
However, remember that no one food is going to be the answer to weight loss – only a combination of effective diet and exercise will really work.

COMBATING STRESS AND CALORIES!

Healthy calorie intake

A 20-year-old woman who weighs 58kg needs 2,200 calories a day to keep her weight constant. She'd need more calories if she were pregnant or breastfeeding, and less if she were trying to lose weight.

One kilogram of fat contains approximately 7,700 calories, so to lose half a kilo a week, a person should take in approximately 3,850 fewer calories a week. This can be done by reducing the daily intake by 550 calories a day (550 times seven days will provide a deficit of 3,850 calories a week). So, to lose one kilo a week, you need to eat 1,100 calories a day less than you normally do.

If this seems impossible, remember that your daily exercise and activity also contribute significantly to burning calories. So there's no need to starve yourself! The lowest daily recommended number of calories for a woman is 1,200 (1,600 for a man), unless you're on a medically-supervised, very low-calorie regime, which may have a daily limit of 500–800 calories.

Calories and kilojoules

Energy is expressed as calories or kilocalories. More recently, the units of energy have been changed to kilojoules. There are 4.2 kilojoules in one kilocalorie. For example, someone eating 2,000 kilocalories a day would be consuming 8,400 kilojoules.

The energy value of a food indicates its value to the body as a fuel. We need energy to maintain the basic processes of life at rest – that is, to keep us ticking over – plus energy for keeping active. Body weight is also an important factor in determining how much energy you need, since if you're heavier you'll need more to sustain you and keep you on the move.

Fat is the most energy-dense food, followed by alcohol, protein and carbohydrate. For example, one double whisky has about twice as many

COMBATING STRESS AND CALORIES!

calories as a glass of soft drink. A glass of full-fat milk has about twice the calories as a glass of soft drink or of skimmed milk. Micronutrients – vitamins and minerals – have virtually no energy value.

The word 'energy' has been used here in the nutritional sense of 'provider of fuel' and not in the sense of providing zest and vitality. High-energy foods do not necessarily affect how we feel. Foods are sometimes promoted as mood-changers on the basis of their energy value, but this is simply playing on the double-meaning of 'energy'.

Activity

Active rest day

Move it or lose it! Use the stairs, take walking breaks, leave your car at home... whatever you do, keep moving.

TOP TIP

◆ Consider working one-on-one with a personal trainer. Get a customised fitness tutorial from a certified expert, who can monitor your movements and point you in the right direction.

MYTH: Exercise makes you eat more.
FACT: Research has shown that after 20 minutes of exercise people ate no more than those who had done nothing. The only difference was that those who had exercised thought the food tasted better.

COMBATING STRESS AND CALORIES!

Get off and stay off

Going on a drastic diet is hard work. It's easy to lose weight, but then just as easy to return to old eating patterns. You feel a failure, so you go on a diet again and again... You become a slave to dieting.

Rather than worry about the mirror and the scales, let's think about your lifestyle and your health. Being healthy doesn't mean you have to be a size 8 or a size 10. It means feeling good physically and emotionally, and having energy and vitality to enjoy every day. It isn't difficult to lead a healthy lifestyle, feel great and still have room for the occasional treat.

Why are you overweight?

During the last 50 years, the amount of food we eat has decreased, while our average body weight has gone up. There's a very simple explanation for this – we've become less active. We watch more television, spend more time in front of computers, and use cars instead of walking or cycling. So we burn up far fewer calories than our parents' generation did.

What we weigh depends on a simple balance: the calories we consume versus the calories we burn. Or, put more simply, food versus activity and exercise. You may not seem to eat very much, but if you're a couch potato, you still end up piling on the weight.

What can you do about it?

Most people's idea of a diet is to go on a hunger-driven eating plan, which forbids all their favourite foods. If you stick to it, you'll probably lose weight, but at what cost? It's impossible to stick to for long, so when you do eventually abandon the diet all those kilos pile back on even faster than they went away.

COMBATING STRESS AND CALORIES!

116

The benefits of exercise

With experience and professional guidance, you learn that the only way to diet sensibly is to follow a healthy, balanced diet with lots of fresh fruit and vegetables, not much fat, and moderation in all things.

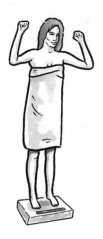

Almost anyone can lose weight – the trick is to keep it off. But the process doesn't have to be unpleasant. Exercise is the key. It will help to shape a fitter and more energetic body, which means you'll have a more enjoyable lifestyle. The good news is that the longer you can maintain your weight loss, the less effort it takes.

Activity

Cardio 23-minute power walk

Every day you're becoming fitter, more energised and better able to cope with what life throws at you. While you're out on your power walk, think about what this walk means to you. Try walking a little further today, making sure your legs are really striding out. Feel them getting firmer as you walk with real purpose.

A thorough stretch is much needed now, so get comfortable and ease yourself into every stretch while breathing deeply for a really relaxing effect.

COMBATING STRESS AND CALORIES!

Are you keeping up? Do you need some help? If you've not already subscribed, why not try the daily text messaging service for extra encouragement and support.
Just text 'Body Idol 41' to 80881 now.

Each set of messages costs £1.50. Please see page xiv for full terms and conditions.

Weight-loss tips

Follow these key weight-loss strategies for success.

Buy books or magazines related to nutrition or exercise

◆ Opt for credible sources of information – you don't want to get bogged down with confusing, inaccurate or contradictory facts. Don't believe everything you read in glossy publications or the tabloid press. Instead, check the facts with a health and fitness professional.

Your personal recording diary

◆ Record everything you eat and drink and how much you exercise in your personal recording dairy – it's a great way to monitor your progress and keep you motivated.

◆ Weigh yourself once a week or fortnight. Use your weigh-in as a guide for you to modify your eating patterns if you're becoming a bit careless, or to reconsider your exercise patterns. Record this information in your diary.

Looking good

◆ Keep a picture of yourself looking good and feeling happy. You might want to choose a photo of you when you were slimmer as a target to reach to inspire you! Put the picture in a prominent place over your bed, on the fridge door or on the mirror.

Stay healthy at home

◆ Don't keep lots of high-fat foods in the house. This might be difficult if you've got children at home, but there's no harm in instilling healthy eating habits at an early age. Their health counts too!

COMBATING STRESS AND CALORIES!

- Keep lots of healthy foods in the house. Stock up on delicious and nutritious fruit and vegetables. Keep your fridge full of healthy options and you'll soon be craving these rather than the high-fat choices that do nothing for your thighs!
- Don't go out to restaurants as much. If you do love eating out, you can eat healthily. Go easy on the alcohol, avoid fried or high-fat choices and sauces, have smaller portions, and choose fruit salad or a sorbet for dessert.

Exercise, exercise, exercise

- Keep up the exercise! You'll be burning an average of 2,500 calories every week, which shows just how important it is to keep exercising – even when you reach your target weight.
- Spend more time with friends who exercise – their active lifestyles can really encourage you and you can arrange fun, active outings together.

It's simple!

Losing weight is simple, which is not to say that it's necessarily easy! If you're having a hard time keeping the weight off, pick five of the tips listed above and incorporate them into your life. Yes – weight loss is an individual thing, but using tested and proven strategies can only stack the odds in your favour.

Activity

Light cardio exercise

Today is an extra day of light cardio exercise. Choose an activity you like and do it for at least 20 minutes at a medium pace – a little out of your comfort zone but not a killer. It can be anything that gets your heart rate up – walking, swimming, cycling, dancing, etc.

COMBATING STRESS AND CALORIES!

Your notes

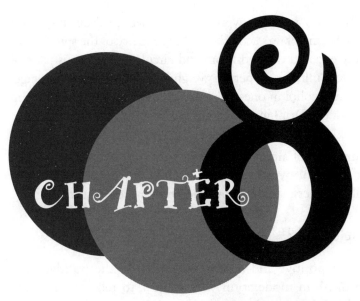

CHAPTER 8

**CHANGE YOUR
DRINKING HABITS**

What's your poison?

Alcohol can be harmless and enjoyable, if it's used responsibly. It comes in different varieties, of course. Beer and ale (4–7% alcohol), wine and champagne (9–14%) and spirits (40–50%) are the most common kinds.

But alcohol is also a sedative hypnotic – a powerful drug. It's also a depressant. It slows the brain's activities and the activity of the spinal cord. Alcohol rapidly enters the bloodstream and circulates to various parts of the body in a few minutes. A person weighing 68kg could, on average, drink one unit of alcohol in one-and-a-half hours without accumulating alcohol in the blood. Drinking any faster would mean they get drunk.

Even small amounts of alcohol can reduce co-ordination, slow down reflexes and lead to overconfidence. Drinking can also result in accidents, falls, sickness, fires, lost productivity and even suicide.

Why do people drink?

People drink for positive and negative reasons. On the positive side, people often drink in moderation with a meal, to relax with family and friends, in religious ceremonies, to celebrate and for medical purposes. Most of the time, this kind of drinking isn't abused.

Negative reasons for drinking are to escape from family problems, as a 'cure' for fears or problems, to block out painful feelings and as a substitute for close relationships. Drinking too much can leave a sense of guilt, which may lead to more drinking. This kind of drinking is often abused. Unfortunately, drinking doesn't solve problems – it just makes matters worse.

When you drink, remember that alcohol is a drug that's potentially addictive. Whenever you drink, you should ask yourself if the alcohol is doing more good than harm. And if you choose not to drink, you'll be in good company.

Activity

Cardio 24-minute power walk

Increase your walk time by an extra minute today. Take big strides and really use your arms to resist the air around them. Smile to yourself and give yourself a pat on the back for keeping up this level of intensity.

Stretch out those tired legs twice today – you'll need it. As you stretch, think about the effort you've made. If you honestly could have done more, make that your goal for your next walk.

'He that takes medicine and neglects diet, wastes the skill of the physician.' Chinese proverb

TOP TIP

◆ Stock up on dried fruit. Dried fruit is low in fat and high in fibre. A good handful also counts as one of your fruit servings for the day.

MYTH: You shouldn't start resistance exercises until you've lost most of your planned weight because it will slow down your fat loss or trap your fat in the muscle.
FACT: Resistance training is vital to a weight-loss programme because it burns more calories and it tones your muscles. Start resistance training immediately.

CHANGE YOUR DRINKING HABITS

How alcohol affects your body

Alcohol is a drug. It affects the way you feel and affects all parts of your body.

Diet Heavy drinkers often neglect their diet, which can lead to vitamin deficiencies.

Brain and central nervous system Alcohol impairs judgement, memory, concentration and co-ordination, as well inducing extreme mood swings and emotional outbursts. Long-term drinking can result in permanent brain damage – the brain tissue is reduced and ventricles increase in size.

Heart The heart can be affected by the vitamin deficiencies caused by a neglected diet. The pumping action of the heart weakens, resulting in heart failure.

Lungs High quantities of alcohol can make you stop breathing, then kill you. Your lungs also have a lowered resistance to infection.

Liver Alcohol can seriously damage the liver. Frequent, large amounts of alcohol in the blood cause liver cells to die and prevent the liver from working efficiently. This disease is called cirrhosis. If a healthy person drinks moderately, the damaged liver tissue has time to repair itself. Two-thirds of cases of liver cirrhosis are caused by alcohol.

Intestines Chronic drinking may result in inflammation, ulcers and cancer of the intestines and colon. Nausea, diarrhoea, vomiting, sweating and loss of appetite are common. Alcohol impairs the small intestine's ability to process nutrients and vitamins.

Reproductive organs Your sex life can be harmed by alcohol, as it depresses nerve impulses. In men, it can cause impotence and infertility. Heavy drinking during pregnancy can harm the foetus. The baby, when born, may be very small and could have reduced intelligence and facial deformities. This is called foetal alcohol syndrome. Women also have a high risk of developing breast cancer.

Eyes Drinking too much can cause red eyes and poor vision.

Ears Alcohol diminishes the ability to distinguish between sounds and know the direction they're coming from.

Mouth Alcohol slurs speech and dulls taste and smell, which often reduces appetite.

Throat Heavy drinking can cause irritation and damage to the lining of the oesophagus, which can cause severe vomiting, haemorrhaging, pain and difficulty swallowing.

Bones Alcohol interferes with the body's ability to absorb calcium resulting in osteoporosis, which means bones become weak, brittle and thinner.

Skin Alcohol causes small blood vessels in the skin to widen, allowing more blood to flow close to the skin's surface. This produces a flushed skin colour.

Weight Heavy drinking can cause a serious weight problem due to alcohol's high simple carbohydrate content.

Activity

Mobility exercises/toning and strength

You'll increase your number of sets today, so take at least 45 seconds to rest between each exercise. Mobilise your shoulders, neck, waist and hips before you start today's toning work, then do every exercise slowly and with control. Feel your muscles working and concentrate on keeping the rest of your body stable.

1. Floor arm dips: 2 sets of 10 reps
2. Modified floor press ups: 2 sets of 10 reps
3. Curls ups: 2 sets of 10 reps
4. Chair leg squats: 2 sets of 10 reps

Remember to stretch afterwards!

CHANGE YOUR DRINKING HABITS

Don't do drunk

Most people enjoy the occasional alcoholic drink, whether it's a celebratory glass of champagne or a glass of wine with a meal out.

There's no need to give up alcohol just because you think it's bad. The daily recommended limit is two units for women and three for men (14 units a week for women and 21 units for men).

A unit of alcohol is equal to 10g of alcohol. Here's the unit quantity for some popular drinks.

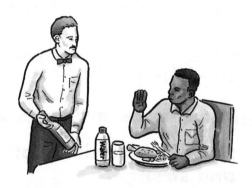

Drink	Number of units
1 small sherry	1
1 glass of wine	1
1 measure of spirit	1
1 pint of beer	2
1 pint of cider	2–4 (depending on strength)
1 bottle of wine	7
1 bottle of vodka	32

Activity

Active rest day

Be sure to move around today. Walk whenever you can and stand up every so often to stretch out your limbs.

TOP TIP

Making just a few changes to your kitchen shelves can really help you to lose weight. Here's what to do.

- Replace corn, coconut or palm oil with olive oil.
- Change white bread to wholewheat.
- Trade in those fatty meats like salami and replace with tinned tuna, sliced turkey/chicken breast or lean roast beef.
- Change from drinking whole milk to fat-free milk or low-fat soya milk. If you find this hard, try semi-skimmed first before you switch to fat-free.

MYTH: Going to a gym is the only way to get fit.
FACT: Any movement is good. You can fit a considerable amount of physical activity into your life by doing things you enjoy. Dance, ride a bike or take a brisk walk on a nature trail. Plan a home workout using a fitness video or DVD. Lift some hand weights or water jugs while watching TV. It all counts. And if you're short of time, break it down. Walk for 10 minutes, three times a day, and you'll still get the health benefits of a 30-minute walk every day.

CHANGE YOUR DRINKING HABITS

Tips for moderate drinking

If you enjoy drinking but are worried about how much or how often you're doing it, try the following tips to encourage moderate drinking.

♦ Always measure your drinks so you know exactly how much you're drinking.

♦ Keep track of how many drinks you have a day. Try to keep this within the recommended daily and weekly allowances.

♦ Before going somewhere where you'll be drinking, decide how much you're going to drink. Make sure that the amount you drink won't make you so drunk that you won't be able to stick to your decision! Remember, a moderate drinker is one who sees alcohol as a drink to enjoy, not as a coping mechanism or as a way to get drunk.

♦ Tell people that you're trying to cut down so that they won't offer you more than you want.

♦ Throughout the evening, alternate your drinks. Start with your favourite soft drink or water then have an alcoholic drink, then a soft one again.

♦ Don't have more than one alcoholic drink an hour. This will help you stay sober and in control.

♦ In a social situation, where people are drinking, always have a drink in your hand. If you've got a soft drink, people will be less likely to offer you an alcoholic one.

♦ Never drink alcohol on an empty stomach.

♦ Avoid being with people who drink to get drunk and who will insist that you do the same.

- Plan how you're going to deal with people who put you under pressure to get drunk. Role play the situation in advance with a supportive friend.

- Build small treats and relaxing things into every day of the week. Try to escape from the thinking process which says 'I deserve to go out and get drunk.'

- Develop some ongoing activities that you enjoy and that don't involve alcohol.

> **MYTH:** You burn more fat if you exercise on an empty stomach.
> **FACT:** Exercising on an empty stomach doesn't affect how you lose weight. In fact, it may hinder weight loss if you don't have the energy to exercise. You should at least drink a glass of juice before your workout if you're exercising in the morning.

Activity Cardio 25-minute power walk

Another day, another minute. Go for it and enjoy the extra time to yourself. Don't be tempted to shuffle along, but pick up your feet and stride out. Get some oxygen inside you and start to feel your body come alive. Feel good, knowing that you're building a healthier body to fend off illness and feeling down.

The harder you exercise the more valuable stretching becomes – so don't miss out – do them now!

Food quiz

No sweat today – just fun, knowledge and health! Enjoy this quiz, but don't peek ahead at the answers. The idea is to learn by thinking through the choices, so the answers are in tomorrow's programme. Good luck!

1. What does a substantial, balanced breakfast do?
a. Leaves you groggier all morning, but helps lose some weight, so the trade off is a personal choice. ☐
b. Makes you lose weight. ☐
c. Double bonus: lose weight, livens the whole morning. ☐
d. Who could eat before midday? ☐

2. Which should you choose – margarine or butter?
a. Neither is harmful. Eat them interchangeably and moderately. ☐
b. Both are unhealthy. Eat neither. ☐
c. Restrict yourself to the softer tub versions of either. ☐
d. As long as they aren't carbs, it doesn't really matter. ☐

3. How safe are beef burgers in relation to ecoli and mad cow disease?
a. Beef burgers are safe when cooked until thoroughly brown in the middle and the juices run clear. ☐
b. They're unsafe when pink in the middle. ☐
c. You must use a meat thermometer to determine their safety. ☐
d. If the outside is partly charred and the burger is still hot, it's safe. ☐
e. Don't worry about ecoli – the real risk is mad cow disease. ☐
f. Don't worry about ecoli or mad cow disease – the biggest danger is the saturated fat in the burger. ☐

4. What's the best way to sweeten your cereal and tea, etc?
a. Aspartame. ☐
b. Table sugar. ☐
c. Brown sugar, molasses, honey, corn syrup, saccharin. ☐
d. Fructose, glucose … the sugars ending in 'ose'. ☐

5. What changes are needed to make the Atkins diet safe and effective in the long term for the general population?

a. None. Recent research has proved that it's safe and effective. ☐

b. Saturated and trans fats, i.e. meat, cheese, margarine, butter, dairy, etc. need to be greatly reduced. ☐

c. Wholegrain bread and pasta needs adding. ☐

d. If it was made safe and effective, it wouldn't be the Atkins diet any more. ☐

6. How healthy is chocolate?

a. It's high in antioxidants, which help prevent disease. Moderate amounts of chocolate will help your health. ☐

b. Its fat content does more harm than its antioxidants do good, so every little bit hurts. ☐

c. As long as your weight is under control, chocolate's calorie count isn't an issue. Enjoy and reap the benefits of the antioxidants. ☐

d. Only dark chocolate with no milk has effective antioxidants. Antioxidants haven't been proven beneficial anyway and few chocolates have no milk. So avoid chocolate. ☐

7. Which kills more people in Britain – cigarettes or obesity?

a. Obesity. ☐

b. Cigarettes. ☐

c. Currently cigarettes, with obesity catching up and about to take over within a year or two. ☐

d. Heart disease and cancer. ☐

Activity

Active rest day

Take some time to relax, but not for the whole day! Think of your body as an efficient watch with all its parts working in unison to keep the watch ticking over smoothly, with precise accuracy. Your body also needs constant movement to keep in tip-top, working condition.

CHANGE YOUR DRINKING HABITS

Food quiz answers

Here are the answers from yesterday's food quiz:

1. The answer is c. If your answer was d, just wait until you start eating more in the morning and less in the evening. Your health, weight, alertness, memory, attention span and physical performance will all improve.

2. The answer is b. Give up both and use olive or sunflower oil instead. Trans fats in margarine aren't good for us and butter is a saturated fat bomb.

3. The best answer is f in the long term, or c in the short term. Ground meat must reach 160 degrees in its thickest part to kill food poisoning bacteria, and that can mean anywhere from pink to brown. Charred meat can cause cancer, and mad cow disease is less of a risk than lightning.

4. The answer is a. Aspartame is safe, non-fattening and avoids the aftertaste of saccharin (which is also safe). The other options are just sugar in different guises, and high-fructose corn syrup is being criticised as a hazardous invention of the late 20th century. (IBS cramps could be the result of too much high fructose corn syrup.) Aspartame's only risk is to people who have phenylketonuria (PKU), who would know if they have it.

5. The answer is d. Recent tests, funded by Atkins, surprised the medical field by lowering cholesterol and triglycerides and confirmed that people can lose weight quickly initially with the Atkins diet. But very few people stick with it, which is good because overwhelming evidence still proves that it's harmful in the long term. We need carbs, and even the Atkins team now admits that you should cut down on the fat. Low carb is still hype, unless you're diabetic or pre-diabetic.

6. The best answer is d. Only dark chocolate raises blood stream antioxidants. Antioxidants haven't been proven to prevent disease and any form of chocolate contains saturated and trans fats. Treat chocolate as the rare, 'sinful' treat that it is.

7. The best answer is c. The final cause of death is often d, but so many of the heart attacks and cancer are caused by c. Either way, our choices are killing us.

Activity

Cardio 26-minute power walk

Watch out for your posture. Are you still making a real effort to keep yourself upright and tucked in? Are you standing and walking tall and proud, lifting your ribcage and breathing well? Get your shoulders back and down and walk with a real sense of purpose.

Remember to counteract your workout with some stretching afterwards.

MYTH: An apple a day keeps the doctor away.
FACT: People who eat temperate fruit such as apples (as opposed to tropical fruit) have a lower risk of heart disease. Apples are part of the carbohydrate group that has a low glycaemic index and, therefore, only slightly raise blood-sugar levels.

CHANGE YOUR DRINKING HABITS

Testing, testing 1, 2, 3

It's now been over six weeks since you embarked on the *Body Idol* programme. You've gone from doing nothing to something. During this time, you've experienced many beneficial changes. You feel and look different for all the right reasons – a much better person on the inside and out.

A great way to measure your achievements is not only by how well your clothes fit and how you look in the mirror, but by retesting your overall condition. Just as you did at the start of this programme, run through the tests in Appendix 3. Record your results as you did before, then follow up with your total scores. You'll be surprised, so give it a go!

'Leave your drugs in the chemist's pot if you can heal the patient with food.' Hippocrates, Greek physician

 TOP TIP 1

♦ If you think you need a very sweet treat every night, try to strike a balance with healthy choices. Compromise with low-fat ice cream and fruit or go for fruit with a topping of whipped cream.

 TOP TIP 2

♦ Remember: you can do it! You can't see it when you lower your cholesterol or reduce your risk of diabetes, but that doesn't mean you aren't doing yourself a huge favour. A longer, healthier life is definitely worth the exercise.

CHANGE YOUR DRINKING HABITS

Activity

Mobility exercises/ toning and strength

Warm up beforehand, as a big change happens today. Your floor dips have been replaced with chair dips, making the exercise tougher but more effective. Your body is stronger now and capable of performing more complex exercises. Aim to reach the maximum reps for the day. Do every rep slowly and with full control.

1. Chair/bench arm dips: 1 set of 10 reps

2. Modified floor press ups: 1 set of 12 reps

3. Curls ups: 1 set of 14 reps

4. Abdominal curls: 1 set of 14 reps

5. Chair leg squats: 2 sets of 12 reps

Familiarity can lead to boredom, so try mixing up your stretches a bit more.

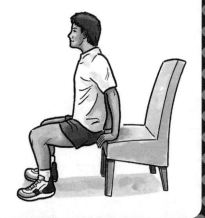

Your notes

CHAPTER 9

SLEEP TIGHT AND STAND STRAIGHT

Sleep test

Now you're mid-way through your life-transforming programme, you must certainly be sleeping like a log. So give the sleep test a go.

Read the statements below. Answer true or false for each one.

	True	False
I feel sleepy during the day, even when I get a good night's sleep.		
I get very irritable when I can't sleep.		
I often wake up at night and have trouble falling back to sleep.		
It usually takes me a long time to fall asleep.		
I often wake up very early and can't fall back to sleep.		
I usually feel achy and stiff when I wake up in the morning.		
I often seem to wake up because of my dreams.		
I sometimes wake up gasping for breath.		
My partner says my snoring keeps them from sleeping.		
I've fallen asleep driving.		

If you answer true for more than three statements, or you're still having sleep difficulties, it's a good idea to discuss your sleep problem with your doctor.

'When diet is wrong, medicine is of no use. When diet is correct, medicine is of no need.' Ancient Ayurvedic proverb

Activity

Cardio 27-minute power walk

Great stuff! Do you realise that, today, you're halfway through your programme? You've done brilliantly. Take time to feel your body's movements and enjoy the feeling of freedom that comes with fitness. Breathe more deeply and breathe out slowly, appreciating the air you're taking in. Enjoy the brisk power walk.

You now know the true value of stretching, but don't think about it – do it!

TOP TIP

- Don't worry about becoming a superstar athlete. Instead, focus on the positive changes you're making to your body and mind. You're relieving stress, building endurance and strengthening your muscles. You're also helping to prevent or delay bone loss and osteoporosis, heart disease, stroke, depression, type two diabetes and some types of cancer.

MYTH: Go for the burn. Remember that saying, 'No pain, no gain'?
FACT: Not true. Exercise shouldn't hurt. A little muscle soreness when you do something new isn't unusual, but soreness doesn't equal pain. You don't need to make your muscles burn to know they're working. If it hurts, stop doing it.

SLEEP TIGHT AND STAND STRAIGHT

The power of posture

Posture is top of the list when you're talking about good health. It's as important as eating properly, exercising, getting a good night's sleep and avoiding potentially harmful substances like alcohol, drugs and tobacco. Good posture is a way of doing things with more energy, less stress and no fatigue. Without good posture, you can't really be physically fit.

Poor posture – how does it happen?

Often, poor posture develops because of accidents or falls. However bad posture can also develop from environmental factors or bad habits. This means that you control it.

Today, posture-related problems are increasing because:

◆ We watch more television than previous generations.
◆ We are increasingly becoming an electronic society, with more and more people working at sedentary desk jobs or sitting in front of computer terminals.
◆ More and more cars are crowding our roads, resulting in accidents and injuries.
◆ We drive in cars with poorly designed seats.

In most cases, poor posture results from a combination of several factors, which can include:

◆ Accidents, injuries and falls
◆ Poor sleep support (the wrong mattress)
◆ Excessive weight
◆ Visual or emotional difficulties
◆ Foot problems or unsuitable shoes
◆ Weak muscles or muscle imbalance
◆ Careless sitting, standing and/or sleeping habits
◆ Negative self image
◆ Occupational stress
◆ Poorly designed workspaces.

SLEEP TIGHT AND STAND STRAIGHT

TOP TIP 1

♦ Cut back on or cut out high-calorie drinks such as cola, lemonade, sweet tea, etc. If you drink two cans of soft drink every day, switch to the diet version or eliminate them completely. From just this one change you could lose up to 11kg in a year. Now that's worth it!

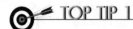
Active rest day

Get off your bum and get active. How about tidying that cupboard you've been meaning to do since the year dot?! Clear out that wardrobe of old clothes that don't fit you since you've lost weight. You'll free up that much-needed space and the charity shop will love you for it.

TOP TIP 2

♦ If you go to a fitness centre, avoid the hard-bodied athletes as you might feel intimidated. But don't hide out alone – hang out with people who are at a similar level of fitness, where you'll feel on more equal ground.

MYTH: Eating most of your calories in the evening promotes weight gain.
FACT: It doesn't matter when you eat them – you gain weight when you eat more calories than you burn off. But mindless munching in front of the TV at night can push calorie intake over the top.

SLEEP TIGHT AND STAND STRAIGHT

Test for posture problems

The wall test

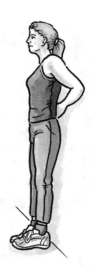

1 Stand with the back of your head touching the wall and your heels 15cm from the skirting board.
2 With your buttocks touching the wall, check the distance between your lower back and the wall with your hand, and your neck and the wall.

If you can get your body between 2.5–5cm from the wall at the lower back and 5cm from the wall at the neck, you're close to having excellent posture. If you can't achieve this, your posture may need professional attention from a chiropractor to restore the normal curves of your spine.

The mirror test

Front view

Stand facing a full-length mirror. For good posture, check that the following are true of you.

1 Your shoulders are level.
2 Your head is straight.
3 The spaces between your arms and sides seem equal.
4 Your hips are level.
5 Your kneecaps face straight ahead
6 Your ankles are straight.

SLEEP TIGHT AND STAND STRAIGHT

Side view

This is much easier to do with somebody helping you or by taking a photo. Stand sideways on to a full-length mirror and check the following.

1 Your head is erect, not slumping forward or backwards.
2 Your chin is parallel to the floor, not tilting up or down.
3 Your shoulders are in line with your arms, not drooping forward or pulled back.
4 Your stomach is flat.
5 Your knees are straight.
6 Your lower back has a slightly forward curve (not too flat or not curved forward too much, creating a hollow back).

Activity

Cardio 28-minute power walk

This daily walk helps you to stay on the right track, by increasing your daily activity level. It's also creating a positive new habit, which you can see and feel is doing you good. During your walk today, get in touch with your body, to take stock of what's happening to your posture and breathing. Enjoy the oxygen stimulating and helping to energise your entire body.

After your energetic power walk, your legs really need some good stretching. Spend a little more time on them today and hold each stretch for longer than usual. Feel yourself easing and relaxing your muscles. Try stretching a little further with every out breath, but be careful not to force it.

SLEEP TIGHT AND STAND STRAIGHT

Top tips to improve your posture

◆ **Standing** Hold your head high, with your chin firmly forward, shoulders back, chest out and stomach tucked in to increase your balance. If you stand all day in a job, rest one foot on a stool or take breaks to get off your feet for a while.

◆ **Sitting** Use a chair with a firm low-back support. Keep your desk or table top at elbow height, so that when your forearms are on the table, your arms form a near-perfect right angle (90 degrees). Adjust the chair or use a footrest to keep pressure off the back of your legs and keep your knees a little higher than your hips. Get up and stretch frequently – every hour if you sit for long stretches. Don't sit on a fat wallet or mobile phone – it can cause hip imbalances!

◆ **Working on a computer** Take a one or two minute breaks every 20 minutes when working at a computer screen. Keep the screen 15 degrees below eye level. Put reference materials on a copy stand close to the terminal and at the same level.

◆ **Sitting in the car** Move the seat forward so that your knees are higher than your hips. Put a small pillow or cushion in the small of your back.

◆ **Sleeping** Sleep on your side with your knees bent and head supported by a pillow, to make your head level with your spine. Alternatively, sleep on your back, avoiding thick pillows. Use a small pillow under your neck instead. Don't sleep on your stomach.

◆ **Lifting** Let your legs do the work to avoid injury to your lower back. Stand close to the object and, where possible, squat down and straddle it. Grasp the load and slowly lift it by straightening your legs as you stand up. Carry the object close to your body.

◆ **Bending** Never twist from the waist and bend forward at the same time. To lift or reach something on the floor, bend you knees while keeping your back straight.

If you follow these tips, but still feel discomfort and pain when doing specific activities, go and see your doctor or chiropractor periodically for spinal checkups and for a postural evaluation.

SLEEP TIGHT AND STAND STRAIGHT

Activity

Mobility exercises/toning and strength

You're now feeling strong, lean and toned from targeting your body through resistance training. To help you keep up the good work, you're going to increase the number of sets for a couple of exercises.

1. Chair/bench arm dips: 1 set of 10 reps

2. Modified floor press ups: 2 sets of 10 reps

3. Curls ups: 1 set of 15 reps

4. Abdominal curls: 1 set of 15 reps

5. Chair leg squats: 2 sets of 15 reps

Slight soreness after exercise means that you've worked your body to the right intensity. To avoid any real discomfort and stiffness, make sure you don't skip your stretching routine.

TOP TIP

- For those mornings when breakfast at home simply isn't an option, grab a piece of fruit and a wholegrain muffin to enjoy on your way to where you're going.

SLEEP TIGHT AND STAND STRAIGHT

145

Energy systems

Adenosine triphosphate (ATP)

The food we eat, in the form of carbohydrates, fats and proteins, is used as fuel for reactions in our body. To make best use of these fuels in our muscles, the body converts them to adenosine tri-phosphate (ATP). There are essentially two ways of producing ATP: aerobically and anaerobically. 'Aerobic' means 'with oxygen', while 'anaerobic' means 'without oxygen'.

Aerobic activity

For low-intensity activities, such as sleeping, working and jogging – and more intense activities carried out over a period of time, such as marathon running – ATP is mainly produced aerobically.

ATP is supplied relatively slowly during the aerobic processes, therefore a person's activity is also relatively slow. As long as there is a continual supply of fuel (e.g. fats and carbohydrates stored in the body) and oxygen, aerobic activities can continue for long periods.

Anaerobic activity

For more explosive movements, such as sprinting or jumping, ATP is needed at a faster rate and can be supplied anaerobically. There are two ways in which the body produces energy anaerobically:

1. The muscles can use stores of ATP (or a similar compound called phosphocreatine, which is already stored in the muscles).
2. The muscles will use the lactate anaerobic system (so called because lactic acid is a by-product). This anaerobic process can't carry on indefinitely as the stores of ATP or phosphocreatine become depleted, and lactic acid builds up within the muscles, causing muscle pain and tiredness.

SLEEP TIGHT AND STAND STRAIGHT

Energy systems working together

During exercise, both aerobic and anaerobic systems work together. However, the proportion of ATP supplied from each process varies according to the intensity and length of exercise. For example, 100m sprinters will mainly use the anaerobic system, an 800-metre runner will use both anaerobic and aerobic systems, while a long-distance runner will get most of their energy from aerobic processes.

Activity

Active rest day

Being more active, even if you're not exercising, can help you lose weight. Every movement counts. So, get moving. For example, if you weigh 70kg and go and cut the grass for 30 minutes (with a manual non-motorised lawn mower of course!) you burn about 175 an calories. Similarly, if you spend an hour washing and waxing your car, you'll burn off an amazing 300–400 calories.

TOP TIP 1

◆ Have a fruit juice or tomato juice instead of a diet soft drink for your afternoon drink.

TOP TIP 2

◆ If you feel you've reached a plateau and/or are bored, don't give up – this is a natural part of working out. Make sure you vary the exercises, sets, repetitions and order of your workout. Continually search for new ways of making your routine fun and exciting.

SLEEP TIGHT AND STAND STRAIGHT

A balancing act

We take balance for granted. Just think, without it you'd fall over time and time again. Worse still, you could cause yourself a nasty injury or even knock yourself out. This simple test for balance is an ideal way to check how even your keel is!

The stork test

1. Stand comfortably on both feet.
2. Put your hands on your hips.
3. Lift one leg and place the toes of that foot against the knee of the other leg.
4. Raise your heel and stand on your toes.
5. Start counting
6. Balance for as long as possible without letting the heel touch the ground or the other foot move away from the knee.
7. Record how long you can balance for.
8. Repeat the test with the other leg.

How well did you do?

Scores for men and women	Excellent	Above average	Average	Below average	Poor
Duration	>30 secs	23–30 secs	16–22 secs	10–15 secs	<10 secs

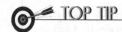

TOP TIP

♦ Take fitness breaks instead of coffee breaks. Spend the time taking a 15-minute walk.

SLEEP TIGHT AND STAND STRAIGHT

Activity

Cardio 29-minute power walk

Six weeks ago just the thought of doing 10 minutes of walking may have been a daunting prospect. Now you're up to 29 minutes – fantastic! You're now feeling full of zest, vim and vigour. Keep it going – get out there today and push yourself a little harder. Really get your arms pumping and take long, fast strides with your legs. Work up a good sweat and enjoy the fact that it's for your own good.

Now do some stretching. Any sign of doing the 'splits' yet? Can you get one leg behind your head? If you can, that's very impressive and illustrates supreme flexibility. If you can't, don't worry, as that degree of suppleness takes hours and years of daily stretching! But you should be able to bend down and reach things much more easily than when you first started. That's a sign that your flexibility is improving and that you've been disciplined enough to stretch regularly. Keep it up!

MYTH: If you're overweight, don't let anybody see you eating 'fattening' foods or they'll say, 'Look at that fat person making themselves fatter!'
FACT: They might say that, but they'll be wrong. There's no such thing as 'fattening' food, just the calories you eat. And people don't know how many calories you've eaten or will eat that day. In France, the average person eats more fat than we Brits do but French people, on average, weigh less than us. Why? Because many French people are trained from childhood to eat what they like of fine foods and savour every bite. This means they rarely feel deprived enough to want to overeat.

SLEEP TIGHT AND STAND STRAIGHT

It's trendy to be bendy

Today, retake the 'flexibility test' from Day 5. How are you progressing with your flexibility and suppleness? Remember, it's essential to warm up before you do the exercises.

The test includes the following exercises:

◆ Sit and reach
◆ Shoulder extension
◆ Forward flexion.

Check your results afterwards. If they weren't great, work a little harder on your stretching exercises to improve your rating when you try the test again.

'The discovery of a new dish confers more happiness on humanity, than the discovery of a new star.' Jean Anthelme Brillat-Savarin, French lawyer and politician

TOP TIP 1

◆ Next time you're feeling wiped out late in the afternoon, forget the cup of coffee and reach for a yoghurt instead. The combination of protein, carbohydrate and fat in a low-fat yoghurt will give you a sense of fullness and well-being that coffee can't match, as well as some vital nutrients. If you haven't eaten in three to four hours, your blood glucose levels are probably dropping, so eating a small amount of nutrient-rich food will give your brain and body a boost.

Activity

Mobility exercises/toning and strength

You're now more in control of your movements. Stay in touch with your muscles as you do every exercise. It really helps to visualise the muscles working. You'll notice that your chair squats have been dropped for now and the static wall squats have been introduced to help you shape your legs even more.

1. Chair/bench arm dips: 2 sets of 10 reps

2. Modified floor press ups: 2 sets of 10 reps

3. Curls ups: 1 set of 18 reps

4. Abdominal curls: 1 set of 18 reps

5. Static wall squats: hold the position for a minimum of 20 seconds (longer if you can)

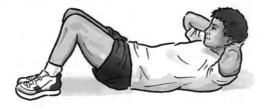

With each stretch, breathe deeply and stretch a little further.

TOP TIP 2

♦ Never underestimate the power of momentum. For starters, take a walk around the block. Don't give up if you feel worn out. Take another walk around the block tomorrow. Eventually, you won't feel worn out any more. That's progress!

SLEEP TIGHT AND STAND STRAIGHT

Your notes

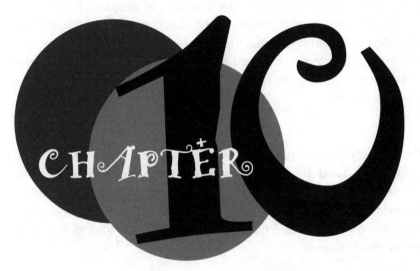

CHAPTER 10

FROM WALKING
TO RUNNING

Get ready to jog

You now have a significant level of fitness and must be feeling that power walking doesn't tax your body as much as it used to. This is a mammoth achievement! This week, you're ready to make the transition from walking to jogging.

Jogging is one of the best forms of exercise for people who want to lose weight, get fit and ensure they don't get heart conditions. Alongside cross-country skiing, jogging – or easy aerobic running – is the best form of exercise to ease pressure on the heart. It develops the circulatory system to gather in and transport more oxygen to various parts of the body.

Although running is a natural activity, it can cause stress to the body if you're not used to it. That's why your programme starts with progressive walking and gradually builds up to jogging. Remember the motto, 'Train, don't strain.' Moderation is key. Too much, too soon, too often, too fast, can create unnecessary stress and delay your physical conditioning.

How far you go isn't that important, as you'll jog at a pace to suit your own comfort zone. First concentrate on being able to jog for the set amount of paces and building up stamina. Then start thinking about picking up speed. Since your heart, lungs and muscles need time to adjust to this new activity, don't run every day.

TOP TIP 1

♦ No energy to exercise? Without exercise, you'll have no energy. It's a vicious cycle. Break the cycle with a walk around the block to boost your energy.

Watch out for signs of overtraining. Tiredness is the first sign. It's followed by pain, tenderness and sweating in the affected area. If you suddenly start sleeping for too long or not enough, it may be due to overtraining or poor nutrition. Pay attention to these symptoms. Your body is trying to tell you to slow down.

TOP TIP 2

♦ Make your activity a regular part of your day, so it becomes a habit.

Activity

Cardio 30-minute power walk

Half an hour of power walking is an amazing achievement. When power walking today, reflect on the positive changes in your life over the last nine weeks. Stay fit and set small, obtainable goals every week. The sense of euphoria from achieving them will mean that you keep looking and feeling as good as you do now.

Afterwards spend some quality stretching time lengthening out those hard-working muscles.

FROM WALKING TO RUNNING

How to jog

As with any other activity, jogging involves a wide variety of individual styles or techniques. Your jogging style should feel comfortable and natural to you. Before you actually give it a try, here is a bit of theory.

Posture

You need to run with your back straight. This helps lessen the stress on your muscles and shifts body weight to the load-bearing bones. Follow this advice even when running up or down hills. Don't lean forward.

Arms

Keep your arms in a comfortable position. When you run, your hands should swing in an arc between your chest line and hip bone. Keep your arms as loose as possible. Don't clench your fists. If you find, for example, that your fingers are swollen or your ring is too tight after a run, it could be because your jogging technique isn't right.

Breathing

Breathe comfortably through your mouth. Follow the 'talk test' – if you can't carry on a conversation while jogging, you're going too fast! Slow down. Conversational jogging is the safest and most efficient way to train.

Legs

Leg movement should be free and easy. A jogger's stride tends to be shorter than a sprinter's. You shouldn't feel uncomfortable while jogging. Proper posture and stride are important, but don't be overly concerned with these – motivation and discipline are just as important!

FROM WALKING TO RUNNING

Feet

It's amazing how many joggers get it wrong! Avoid landing on your toes first. The pressure should be absorbed by your heel. The most efficient way to jog is to land flat-footed or heel first. Roll your foot forward and push yourself into your next stride off the ball of your foot. Listen to your footsteps. If you hear your feet pounding or slapping on the ground you're not doing it right. If you don't hear any pounding, you're doing OK. You're less likely to get injured by jogging silently.

Where you jog

With this jogging style you won't have to worry about the hardness of the pavement. You'll hardly notice whether you're jogging on grass or concrete. To protect your knees and ankles, vary the ground you run on. Pavements are often banked and dip towards the curb. Jogging on this angled surface can cause uneven stress on your legs.

TOP TIP

◆ Focus on positive self-talk. Congratulate yourself every time you take a step towards your goal. Be your own best supporter.

Activity

Active rest day

The key to fitness is not just vigorous activity – it's also moving more during your daily life. How about giving your house or flat a quick once over today for 30 minutes? If you weigh around 70kg, you'll burn about 150 calories.

FROM WALKING TO RUNNING

Drugs are for mugs

Why do people try drugs?

People take drugs to change the way they feel. If they're depressed, they want to be happy. If they're stressed or nervous, they want to relax. By taking drugs, people often think they can change into the person they want to be. The trouble is – it isn't real. They haven't changed their situation – they've only distorted it for a while.

Wanting to fit in Sometimes people take drugs to fit in and to cover-up their insecurities. They don't think about how drugs could isolate them from friends or family. They forget to look past that one party to see how things could turn out. Or they just don't notice the people around them who aren't using drugs.

Needing to escape or relax Some drug-takers drink or take drugs to avoid dealing with their problems or reaching out for help. Unfortunately, the problems are still there when they come down, and they'll still have to deal with them when they're feeling rough, guilty and not thinking straight.

Boredom Lots of people turn to drugs for excitement because they say there's nothing else to do but watch repeats on TV or hang out at the local burger bar. But drugs don't change the situation, and they just might make it worse.

The media says it's cool Despite anti-drug campaigns, the entertainment world still manages to make drugs appear very attractive. But if you're wise, you'll understand that the world on TV and in the papers isn't real, and basing your life on these messages is superficial.

Wanting to seem grown up The reality is that the most adults out there aren't drug users. They're too busy living their lives to bother with drugs.

Wanting to rebel Sometimes people turn to drugs to make a statement against someone else, like their family or society. Taking drugs makes them feel rebellious and more individual. But ultimately, drugs rob people of their independence, because they make them dependent – on drugs and their drug connections.

Wanting to experiment It's human nature to want to experiment. But it's also human nature to avoid things that are obviously bad for you – for example, you wouldn't experiment with jumping off London Bridge! There are a zillion better things than drugs to experiment with – sports, music, dying your hair, etc.

Activity

30-minute cardio power walk/slow jog

Today marks a major change – a distinctive turning point in your quest for greater fitness and well-being. You've been pondering how much easier walking has become and that it's time for another change. This is what you're going to do to take yourself to new heights.

Spend the first 20 minutes of your session power walking at a brisk pace. Then, for the remaining 10 minutes, jog at a slow, steady pace for 30 paces, followed immediately by 100 paces of power walking. Make sure your jogging technique is correct, so refer to Day 57 for guidance.

You'll soon realise that a bit of jogging is slightly harsher on your body than walking. That's why it's essential to do some proper stretching afterwards. Spend a little longer with each muscle group.

FROM WALKING TO RUNNING

Are drugs always bad?

Illegal drugs are always bad. There aren't any benefits from sniffing glue or snorting heroin. But many drugs were developed by doctors to help treat patients with specific medical conditions. And for these people, prescription drugs make sense. Unfortunately, many of these drugs are used illegally by people who don't need them.

What do drugs feel like?

Depending on the drug, many people report feelings like happiness, confidence, serenity or euphoria. In most cases, these feelings are followed by even more powerful ones like depression, anxiety, nausea, guilt, embarrassment, loneliness and wanting more drugs.

Effects of using drugs

Short term

- Every drug is different, but they all interfere with the nervous system's basic functions. Sometimes they alter muscles and how they function.
- Almost all drugs can make it tougher to sleep.
- Some cause major weight gain; others cause unhealthy weight loss and diarrhoea.
- Eyes can become glassy and bloodshot.
- Some drugs, like glue or butane, can kill you immediately. Cocaine, ecstasy and meths can give you a heart attack on the spot.
- Most drugs make your hair and skin much less healthy and many will cause spots on your face and body.
- Smoking marijuana can make your teeth yellow.
- Drugs can interfere with your sexual performance.

Long term

- Using drugs repeatedly for a long period of time can cause lots of medical problems, from lung cancer (marijuana) to liver problems (alcohol) to brain damage (ecstasy, alcohol).
- Depression is a serious problem for many addicts. They may also tell lies, steal money for drugs or become violent.
- Many people who take drugs become physically or mentally addicted. They want more – and they feel like they need more.

Eventually, trying to get drugs becomes the most important thing in their lives, using up all their time, money and energy and really hurting people they're close to.

Can you get addicted even though you only do it once in a while?

Addiction is a process – not a one-off event. Some drugs make users feel so good that they're always searching for that initial high. But they rarely get the feeling they want, so some keep searching and taking more or different drugs.

Meanwhile permanent changes are happening in users' brains – they're starting to get addicted. Using drugs occasionally turns into using drugs a fair amount, which can turn into using drugs a lot. No one knows when the 'chemical switch' goes off in a person's brain or who will get addicted – it's like playing Russian Roulette. The only thing experts do know is that the more you do drugs, the closer you get to addiction.

Activity

Mobility exercises/toning and strength

Today, weights will add another dimension to your resistance exercises to further your body sculpting. You'll be targeting arms, shoulders, the lower stomach, buttocks and legs. Check your technique by studying the descriptions and illustrations carefully before you try these new exercises. Don't forget your warm-up exercises before you start.

1. Weighted arm curls: 1 set of 12 reps
2. Weighted overhead press: 1 set of 12 reps
3. Abdominal reverse curls: 1 set of 20 reps
4. Static wall squats: hold the position for a minimum of 25 seconds (longer if you can)

You'll soon discover that weights challenge your body in a different way, making the exercises that much more intense. It's now vital for you to stretch – so get to it!

FROM WALKING TO RUNNING

Signs and symptoms

Do you or your friends have a drink or drug problem? If you do one or more of the following, the chances are there's a problem:

- Use drugs or alcohol regularly and have to use them to have a good time or cope with everyday life
- Start hanging out with new friends who also do drugs
- Turn up at work drunk or high or skip a meeting to use
- Break plans or show up late, due to getting drunk or high
- Show little interest or drop out altogether from previously enjoyable activities
- Drink or use drugs when alone
- Drive a car while drunk or high, or catch a lift with somebody else who is drunk or high
- Borrow money to buy drugs or alcohol
- Must be looked after when drunk or high to stop them doing things they might regret, like having sex or driving under the influence of drugs or alcohol.

TOP TIP 1

- If you really hate vegetables and love fruit, eat plenty of them. They're just as healthy, especially colourful ones like passion fruit, oranges, mangoes and melons.

TOP TIP 2

- Reframe the way you think about exercise. Begin to think of every workout as a gift you give to yourself instead of just another 'should', 'ought' or 'must'.

TOP TIP 3

- Make healthy eating and physical activities fun! Go out with friends and do physical activities together, and eat the foods you like together too. Be adventurous – try new sports, games and other activities as well as new foods. You'll grow stronger, play longer, and look and feel better.

'Life consists not in holding good cards, but in playing those you hold well.' Josh Billings, American humourist and lecturer

Activity

Active rest day

Gardening is an excellent way to burn some extra calories. If you weight 70kg, you'll burn over 100 calories if you dig around in the garden for 20 minutes.

MYTH: You can change your body shape through dieting.
FACT: People often diet not because they're overweight, but because they're unhappy with their body shape. Sadly they're wasting their time. A pear shape will simply be a smaller pear shape after dieting. The only thing that can help is exercise, which can help streamline certain areas.

FROM WALKING TO RUNNING

Are you keeping up? Do you need some help? If you've not already subscribed, why not try the daily text messaging service for extra encouragement and support.
Just text 'Body Idol 61' to 80881 now.

Each set of messages costs £1.50. Please see page xiv for full terms and conditions.

What happens if you keep using drugs?

Think about how you feel when something good happens – maybe your team wins a game, you get praise for something or you drink a cold lemonade on a hot day – this is the limbic system at work in our brains. This system is primarily responsible for our emotional life; it creates an appetite that drives you to seek those things we enjoy.

The first time someone uses a drug, they experience unnaturally intense feelings of pleasure. Of course, drugs have other effects too: a first-time smoker may cough and feel sick from toxic chemicals in a cigarette or marijuana joint.

The brain starts changing right away as a result of the unnatural flood of neurotransmitters. One of the neurotransmitters playing a major role in addiction is dopamine. Dopamine is similar to adrenaline; it affects brain processes that control movement, emotions and the experience of pleasure and pain. Drugs can bind to dopamine receptors and can either stimulate them or block them. Different drugs have very different actions.

At what stage does somebody become addicted to drugs?

It's not known how many times a person can use a drug without changing their brain and becoming addicted. But their genetic makeup is likely to be a factor. After a certain number of doses, a person's limbic system craves the drug. This craving is made worse because of down regulation.

Without the drug, dopamine levels in the drug abuser's brain are low. The person feels flat, lifeless, depressed. They need drugs just to bring dopamine levels up to normal. To get a high (or dopamine flood), they need even more of the drug – this effect is known as tolerance.

Drug addiction is a disease and leads to long-term changes in the brain. These changes mean that drug users lose their ability to control their drug use.

If drug addiction is a disease, is there a cure?

There's no complete cure for drug addiction, but it is a treatable disease and drug addicts can recover. Drug-addiction therapy is a programme of behaviour change or modification that slowly retrains the brain. Like people with diabetes or heart disease, people being treated for drug addiction learn behavioural changes and often take medication as part of their treatment regime.

Activity

30-minute cardio power walk/slow jog

You'll really progress today by upping your pace – it's 30 minutes of cardio work. Spend the first 20 minutes of your session power walking at a brisk pace. Don't hold back – make sure you really stride out and swing your arms to help keep up the pace. For the remaining 10 minutes, jog slowly and steadily for 40 paces, then immediately do 100 paces of power walking. Keep your breathing nice and steady.

Pay special attention to giving your legs a good, long stretch – they'll need it.

FROM WALKING TO RUNNING

Top 20 benefits of exercise

Everyone exercises for different reasons. But regardless of your motivation, you still get all the benefits. Starting or continuing your exercise programme is much easier if you know some of the positives you'll get from exercise. If you can find even one benefit on the list below, you'll have enough reason to start an exercise programme.

20 top tips

1. Elevates your metabolism so that you burn more calories every day.
2. Increases your aerobic capacity (fitness level). This means that you can go through your day doing more but using up less energy than you normally do. And you'll still have more energy left at the end of the day!
3. Maintains, tones and strengthens your muscles. Also increases your muscular endurance.
4. Decreases your blood pressure.
5. Increases the oxidation (breakdown and use) of fat ('release the grease!').
6. Increases HDL (good) cholesterol.
7. Makes the heart a more efficient pump by increasing stroke volume (the amount of blood pumped by the heart in one contraction).
8. Increases haemoglobin concentration in your blood. Haemoglobin is found in the red blood cells that carry oxygen from the lungs to the rest of the body.
9. Decreases the tendency of the blood to clot in the blood vessels. This is important because small clots travelling in the blood are often the cause of heart attacks and strokes.
10. Increases the strength of the bones.
11. Causes new blood vessels to develop in the heart and other muscles.
12. Enlarges the arteries that supply blood to the heart.
13. Decreases levels of triglycerides (bad fats) in the blood.
14. Improves blood–sugar control.
15. Improves sleep patterns.
16. Increases the efficiency of the digestive system, which may reduce the incidence of colon cancer.

FROM WALKING TO RUNNING

17. Increases the thickness of cartilage in joints, which has a protective effect on the joints.
18. Decreases a woman's risk of developing endometriosis (a gynaecological condition) by 50%.
19. Increases the amount of blood that flows to the skin, making it look and feel healthier.
20. Exercise, in addition to all the physiological and anatomical benefits, just makes you feel GREAT!

Activity

Mobility exercises/toning and strength

You'll add a couple more reps to your exercises today.

Some of the exercises from earlier in the programme have also been included. Maintain good technique and posture throughout each exercise. For a more intensive workout, make sure you don't rest for longer than 45 seconds between each exercise.

1. Weighted arm curls: 1 set of 14 reps
2. Weighted overhead press: 1 set of 14 reps
3. Abdominal curls: 1 set of 15 reps
4. Curls ups: 1 set of 15 reps
5. Abdominal reverse curls: 1 set of 15 reps
6. Chair leg squats: 1 set of 20 reps
7. Static wall squats: hold the position for a minimum of 30 seconds (longer if you can)

Remember to stretch afterwards!

TOP TIP

♦ Don't try to diet on holiday. Instead, try to keep at your present weight. This is realistic, because you can indulge every once in a while, but you can't have a blowout!

FROM WALKING TO RUNNING

Your notes

....

....

....

....

....

....

....

....

....

....

....

....

....

....

....

....

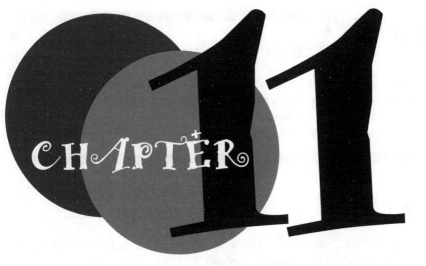

CHAPTER 11

NO TIME TO WASTE

Burn, baby, burn

Most of us have either been obsessed or curious about calories. So how many calories do you use up during the day? Use the chart opposite to calculate the rough number of calories burned during various activities. The chart lists activities in order of effort, starting with the easiest and moving down to the higher-energy one.

Activity

Active rest day

Today, commit yourself to doing something vigorously. For example, vigorously wash the car. Or vigorously weed the garden. Anything counts – as long as it's vigorous!

TOP TIP 1

◆ Use 'light' or low-fat dairy products for snacks or cooking, such as milk, cheese, yoghurt or sour cream. Drink skimmed milk. You'll still get the nutrients and taste but not the fat.

TOP TIP 2

◆ Fight discouragement. If, once in a long while, you blow out a workout because you choose to go out with friends, just accept and enjoy your choice – don't feel guilty. Otherwise, the sense of failure can make it harder to get back on track. Focus on how much progress you've made so far, not on how far you have to go.

Type of exercise	Calories/hour
Sleeping	55
Eating	85
Sewing	85
Knitting	85
Sitting	85
Standing	100
Driving	110
Office work	140
Housework, moderate	160+
Golf with trolley	180
Golf without trolley	240
Gardening, planting	250
Dancing, ballroom	260
Walking, 5km per hour	280
Table tennis	290
Gardening, general	350
Tennis	350+
Water aerobics	400
Skating/rollerblading	420+
Dancing	420+
Aerobics	450+
Bicycling, moderate	450+
Jogging, 8km per hour	500
Gardening, digging	500
Swimming, active	500+
Cross-country ski machine	500+
Rambling/hiking	500+
Step aerobics	550+
Rowing	550+
Power walking	600+
Cycling, indoors	650
Squash	650+
Skipping with rope	700+
Running	700+

NO TIME TO WASTE

Find time for exercise

If you're like most people, finding time for exercise is difficult. Here are 10 top tips to help you.

10 top tips

1. Make exercise a priority. If you're serious about finding time for exercise, then it must be a priority in your life.
2. Block out the same time every day for exercise. This way it becomes part of your daily routine just like brushing your teeth. Guard this time with your life!
3. Exercise first thing in the morning. This is when your time is least likely to get interrupted by other things. Try going to sleep a little earlier and getting up a little earlier so you can fit your exercise in.
4. Turn off the television. The average adult spends 16 hours a week watching TV. You can certainly cut out a few hours a week to make time for exercise.
5. Spend around 30 minutes exercising in your lunch break.
6. Spend some of your reading time exercising on your stair climber or treadmill.
7. Have a chat with a friend or loved one or while walking around the neighbourhood rather than sitting on the sofa.
8. Take a couple of days to write down how you spend your time every day, then plan around this time to fit in exercise.
9. Make your exercise as enjoyable as possible. You'll be much more likely to find time for things you enjoy.
10. Think of ways of building activity into your daily life. It may mean getting off the bus or train stop earlier and walking the rest of the way to where you're going, or simply taking the stairs instead of the lift. Not only is this a great way of burning off more calories, but you can also count it as part of your exercise regime!

'It is not the length of life, but the depth of life.'
Ralph Waldo Emerson, American author, poet and philosopher

Activity

30-minute cardio power walk/slow jog

You've been working very hard over the last 10 weeks. Fitter, stronger, energised, invigorated, confident, persistent, committed and achiever are key words you can use to describe yourself. Let's step up another gear with your aerobic work. Today, the first 20 minutes of your session involve power walking at a brisk pace. Push yourself harder – your fitness will allow it and your body can take it. For the last 10 minutes challenge yourself with a slow, steady jog for 50 paces followed immediately by power walking for 100 paces.

Get down and get stretched!

TOP TIP

♦ Not only does exercise help boost your mood, it also stimulates your muscles, making you feel more alive and connected to your body.

MYTH: If you don't exercise an hour a day, five days a week, you might as well do nothing.
FACT: Don't believe this all-or-nothing approach. The truth is, there are enormous benefits to doing just a little exercise daily. Studies show that a half-hour walk three or more times a week significantly reduces your risk of heart attack and stroke, lowers blood pressure, relieves stress and boosts your energy and immune system.

NO TIME TO WASTE

Beat the biological clock

Ageing is an inevitable process. Every living thing has to age as time passes. Advances in science haven't yet been able to control the signs of ageing, but there are certain lifestyle changes you can make to help you delay the biological clock. Learn to adopt this approach for life!

Five top tips

1. **Eat up to three-quarters of your capacity** When you eat less, you produce fewer free radicals (cell-damaging oxygen molecules), which are known to be the prime players in accelerating the ageing process. Excess calories (in other words, overeating) are the enemies of youth.

2. **Balance your appetite** If you feel really hungry a lot of the time (a sign of excess heat in the body), balance your appetite by eating raw, cooling vegetables like cucumber, celery, cabbage, radish, lettuce and tomatoes, and fruit like watermelon, apple, banana, oranges, grapefruits and pears.

3. **Drink lots of tepid water (10–12 glasses daily), watery soups and vegetable broths** Water plays a number of roles in keeping you healthy. It helps to digest food so you can absorb the nutrients you need. It gives you an important source of minerals like magnesium and calcium. Water also moistens mucous membranes, lubricates the joints and cools the body through perspiration.

4. **Take antioxidants** Take antioxidants every day in the form of vegetable juice or wheatgrass juice. Or take an antioxidant vitamin supplement containing vitamins A, C and E and the mineral selenium.

5. **Keep active** Exercising and keeping active keeps the body strong, supple and healthy. It means you can perform everyday tasks with less effort and with more energy.

NO TIME TO WASTE

Activity

Mobility exercises/toning and strength

Look in the mirror and notice the great changes in your body. Aren't you glad you started this?! Today there's an increase in the number of reps, and some of the exercises you were doing previously are included to give you a more complete toning workout. This'll be tough, but persevere and make sure you warm up first.

1. Chair dips: 1 set of 15 reps

2. Modified floor press ups: 1 set of 15 reps

3. Weighted arm curls: 1 set of 15 reps

4. Weighted overhead press: 1 set of 15 reps

5. Abdominal curls: 1 set of 20 reps

6. Curls ups: 1 set of 20 reps

7. Abdominal reverse curls: 1 set of 20 reps

8. Chair leg squats: 1 set of 20 reps

9. Static wall squats: hold the position for a minimum of 40 seconds (longer if you can)

Remember to stretch out afterwards!

TOP TIP

♦ Moderate exercise distracts you from negative feelings and forces you to concentrate on your breathing, stamina and physical power. By the time you've completed your workout, your negative feelings are likely to be less intense or even replaced by a stronger sense of accomplishment.

NO TIME TO WASTE

Too much pain, no gain

To keep your body healthy, exercise is essential. But working out can do more harm than good if you don't know how to prevent injuries. Here's how to get the most out of your exercise while keeping your body in one piece.

10 top tips for avoiding injury

1. Don't push through pain. Real discomfort is a signal that something's wrong or that you're asking more from a part of your body than it can give right now.
2. Increase your workouts gradually. If you're jogging, don't bump up your pace too fast.
3. Don't run when it's snowing. Although it would improve your stamina it definitely increases your risk of injury.
4. Run on soft, flat surfaces.
5. Alternate hard training days with easy days.
6. Get new running shoes every 800 kilometres. With use, shoes lose their ability to absorb shock.
7. If you pronate (the inside of your foot leans in) or have another alignment problem, you may be able to prevent injury by wearing an over-the-counter shoe insert.
8. Make sure you're getting enough calcium, whether from your diet or from supplements. Stress fractures are 10 times more common in women than in men. Improve your odds of avoiding them by making sure you get enough of the minerals and vitamins crucial to building bone.
9. Women who have irregular periods should be especially concerned about stress fractures. If this applies to you, talk to your doctor.
10. Ankle sprains may be the most common sports injury that isn't caused by overuse. If ankle sprains are a common problem, go and see a physiotherapist. They may recommend some ankle strengthening or lace-up stabilizers. These devices are particularly important if you lack strength, flexibility or good balance, all of which can help you avoid injury.

Activity

Active rest day

Think of ways to fit in some form of activity other than exercise. Why not take a walk on the wild side or on the sedate side? Whichever side you choose, go for a walk today and aim to be active.

TOP TIP 1

◆ Eat the low-cal items on your plate first. Start with salads, veggies and broth soups, and eat meats and carbs last. By the time you get to them, you'll be full enough to be content with smaller portions of the high-calorie choices.

TOP TIP 2

◆ Believe that your uniqueness is important. If all of us looked the same, thought the same and dressed the same, the world would be a boring place. Wear clothes that flatter your shape no matter what size you are. Your uniqueness contributes to the vast and beautiful tapestry of our world and, as such, you are a valuable member of humanity.

MYTH: Exercise keeps you up all night.
FACT: As long as you don't exercise within four hours of your bedtime, the opposite is true. Exercise contributes to a more restful sleep and makes you more alert in your everyday life.

NO TIME TO WASTE

Read on and on...

Today, why not flash some cash and indulge yourself with some reading? Go out and buy five or six health and fitness magazines and increase your knowledge on the subject. Get informed and be informed.

Good magazines

Personal trainer for women
Zest
Health and fitness
Ultrafit
TopSanté

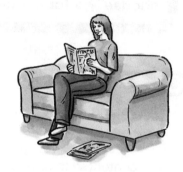

Activity

30-minute cardio power walk/slow jog

Tune in mentally to today's aerobic session as you walk the first 20 minutes of your session at a fast pace. Your next 10 minutes involves the same steady jog for 50 paces but your power walking is reduced to only 50 paces, giving you less recovery time between each interval. Stay focused and give it your best shot.

Now give yourself the stretches you deserve after working up a good, healthy sweat.

'Common sense is in medicine the master workman.' Peter Latham, English physician

TOP TIP 1

◆ Mix different kinds of beans, such as kidney beans, green beans, broad beans or borlotti beans, with some diet salad dressing. Eat this mixed-bean salad for the next few days as a snack or part of your main meals.

TOP TIP 2

◆ If you have children, make time to play with them outside. Set a good example to yourself and your loved ones!

MYTH: By using hand and ankle weights while you jog, you can do strength training and aerobic conditioning at the same time.
FACT: If you want aerobic exercise, then jog. If you want strength, then use resistance exercises. Don't combine them. The momentum that weights generate when you perform aerobic activities can stress tissue and lead to joint and muscle problems.

NO TIME TO WASTE

Get equipped

The minefield of the fitness equipment market can often seem as confusing as choosing a new car. Treadmills, elliptical cross trainers, slam man, dumbbells, barbells, Stairmaster, rowers, recumbent bikes – the list goes on. Why not visit your local sports shop or leisure centre and familiarise yourself with what's on offer? Try some out. You may even end up dragging a machine or two home!

Activity

Mobility exercises/toning and strength

Some new exercises have been added today to target areas of your upper body, waist and stomach. A strong, balanced body equals a more robust body that can cope with everyday life with greater efficiency. Warm up beforehand and study your technique and posture first.

1. Weighted arm extensions: 1 set of 15 reps

2. Weighted side raises: 1 set of 15 reps

3. Weighted front raises: 1 set of 15 reps

4. Bicycles abs: 1 set of 20 reps

5. Hip lifts: 1 set of 20 reps

6. Cross over curls: 1 set of 20 reps

7. Chair leg squats: 1 set of 20 reps

8. Alternate leg lunges: 1 set of 12 reps

NO TIME TO WASTE

'Time is the great physician.' Benjamin Disraeli, England's first and only Jewish Prime Minister

TOP TIP 1

- There are a lot of healthy frozen ready-meals available these days that make mealtimes quick and easy. Choose one low in calories and enjoy with a salad and a glass of low-fat milk.

MYTH: Reduced-fat foods help you lose weight.
FACT: Most diets suggest eating low-fat foods. They can help, but many are bulked out with other ingredients to replace the fat, which means that the calorie count – the crucial factor in determining whether a food will make you put on weight – is barely reduced.

TOP TIP 2

- Whenever you've got an errand to do, park your car as far away as you can handle (or get off the bus a stop early) and walk to the shop. At the shopping centre, if you're driving, park at the farthest end of the car park and walk the length of the centre. Use every opportunity to walk. In the end, it all adds up to better fitness.

MYTH: Popping pills such as 'fat magnets' are an easy option to lose weight.
FACT: Be wary of gimmicks or fads. No magic pill or miracle-working exercise device will help you with your fitness goals. The truth is that you've got to be dedicated and that takes hard work.

NO TIME TO WASTE

Walk and then run

'We are what we repeatedly do. Excellence, then, is not an act, but a habit.' Aristotle, Greek philosopher

Activity

30-minute cardio power walk/slow jog

You'll progress even further today – you're going to reduce your power-walking time and increase the time on your steady jog. Spend the first 18 minutes of your session power walking at your usual brisk pace. Then follow this with 12 minutes of steady jogging for 50 paces combined with 75 paces of power walking. Keep your chest and head high and get those arms working hard and upwards, moving across your body slightly when jogging.

Your front thighs, rear thighs, lower back and calves will need some quality stretching afterwards.

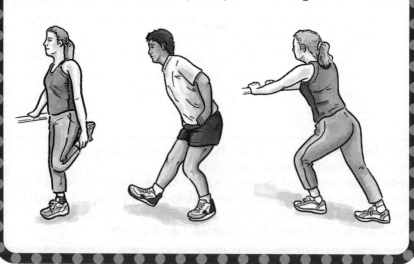

TOP TIP 1

+ Avoid giving yourself a hard time if you take a step backwards or break your fitness resolution. Just brush yourself off and start all over again!

TOP TIP 2

+ Cereal with fruit and fat-free milk makes a good meal at any time of the day and it's very quick and easy to prepare.

TOP TIP 3

+ You shouldn't avoid all fat, because everyone needs some fat in their diet to be healthy. Instead, try to reduce the amount of saturated fats in your diet. These are found in cheese, butter, pastry, biscuits and cakes, and can raise cholesterol and increase the risk of heart disease. Try to replace them with unsaturated fats, which can be found in olive and sunflower oils, nuts and oily fish.

MYTH: You can eat whatever you want if you exercise enough.
FACT: If you eat more calories than you burn off in a day, you'll gain weight. A good fitness regime includes a sensible balance between getting enough exercise and getting the right food.

NO TIME TO WASTE

Your notes

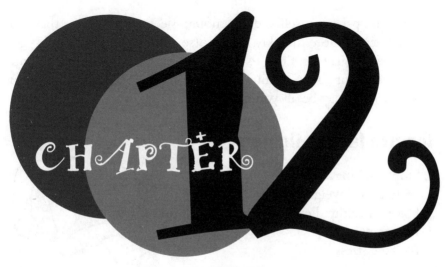

CHAPTER 12

BODY
TRANSFORMATION

Fighting fatigue

We all get tired. An active day that combines working, parenting and housekeeping – or any one of the three – requires a lot of energy. Everyone needs plenty of rest to start afresh the next day, and the next and the next... But if you add the demands of our modern busy lifestyles to the daily mix, you may very quickly find that you're depleting your energy reserves.

If you don't pace yourself and get enough sleep, you'll notice that you become tired more quickly. Or worse than that, you could get exhausted. It may be time to take a long holiday and make some changes to your life. Catching up on your sleep and spending your energy wisely may be all you need to get back on track.

Top five fatigue fighters

1. Stop smoking.
2. Watch your weight.
3. Have a healthy diet.
4. Keep active.
5. Reduce stress.

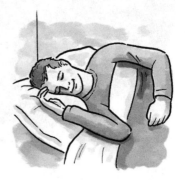

> **MYTH:** Abdominal exercises will flatten your stomach.
> **FACT:** Sorry. Abdominal exercises, such as sit-ups (crunches), are important for strengthening those muscles and improving posture. But muscle is muscle and fat is fat. If you have excess fat in your abdomen, you won't be able to see the muscles, no matter how many crunches you do. There's no such thing as spot reducing – losing weight in one specific area. To lose fat, you need to eat fewer calories than you burn and include aerobic exercise to help shift fat.

BODY TRANSFORMATION

Activity

Active rest day

Have you ever thought about how much time you spend standing in a queue? Although it's annoying to have to wait, it's nice to know that standing in line actually burns calories. If you weigh 70kg, you'll burn 30 calories in 20 minutes. Tap your foot impatiently and you'll probably burn more! You can even use your shopping as weights and exercise whilst in the queue!

What about when gossiping away to a friend on the cordless phone? You still burn a minimal amount of calories, but if you keep on tapping or walk around the house during your chat, you'll burn a whole lot more!

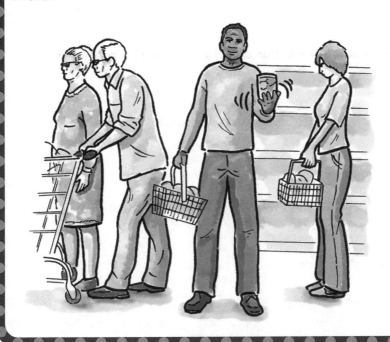

BODY TRANSFORMATION

Are you keeping up? Do you need some help? If you've not already subscribed, why not try the daily text messaging service for extra encouragement and support.
Just text 'Body Idol 71' to 80881 now.

Each set of messages costs £1.50. Please see page xiv for full terms and conditions.

Fit quiz

Find out if your fitness knowledge is up to date with this fit quiz – give it a go! The answers are not until tomorrow!

1. **If you do both weight training and aerobics in the same session, which should come first?**
   - Weight training ☐
   - Aerobics ☐

2. **Exercise gives you an energy boost.**
   - True ☐
   - False ☐

3. **You're stuck with the metabolic rate you're born with.**
   - True ☐
   - False ☐

4. **If you think you've injured a muscle, immediately apply ice.**
   - True ☐
   - False ☐

5. **Which type of exercise is the best way to burn fat?**
   - Vigorous ☐
   - Moderate ☐
   - Doesn't matter ☐

'The sovereign invigorator of the body is exercise, and of all the exercises walking is the best.' Thomas Jefferson, 3rd President of the United States

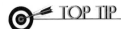

TOP TIP

◆ Avoid situations that put you in temptation's path. As obvious as it sounds, don't stand near the food at parties. By doing this you'll find you eat less.

Activity

30-minute cardio power walk/slow jog

Put your best foot forward first and face this new challenge. 18 minutes of your session involves a strong, fast and hard walk at a good pace. Now pace yourself well for the next 12 minutes as you'll be jogging for 50 paces then power walking for 50 paces.

Afterwards, sit or lie down quietly as you do some deep breathing during stretching. Exert a little more pressure on every stretch if you want to, but take care not to push it too far.

MYTH: Chocolate makes you fat.
FACT: Most diets tell you to avoid chocolate. But scientific studies show that neither chocolate, nor any other individual food, has been implicated as the sole cause of weight gain. Chocolate actually offers some nutritionally beneficial properties such as calcium and protein, but it's also high in sugars and fat so – as with most things – enjoy in moderation!

BODY TRANSFORMATION

Fit quiz answers

1. **Aerobics.** You'll boost circulation and body temperature before working with weights.

2. **True, unless you're tired because of illness, lack of sleep or malnourishment.** Exercise is particularly effective against anxiety and mild depression.

3. **False.** Resting metabolism is largely determined by age (it slows), genes (some people burn faster) and gender (women's rates are usually lower). However, the longer and more intensely you exercise, the higher your metabolic rate, at least temporarily. If you exercise regularly, you'll increase muscle and decrease fat, resulting in a higher metabolism overall.

4. **True.** Apply an ice pack (or even a pack of peas!) for 10 to 20 minutes immediately. Applying heat can increase inflammation during the first couple of days after injury.

5. **It doesn't matter.** If you burn off more calories than you eat over the course of a week or two, you'll start burning fat stores, even through doing normal daily activities.

⊙—≺ TOP TIP

- ◆ After going for a few days without sweets, you'll be able to avoid bingeing on sweet foods.

MYTH: All I need to do to lose weight is go on a diet. **FACT:** Dieting is hard work. Dieting is a constant battle because cells in the brain remember the amount of the fat in the body and keep it constant. When people diet, the brain thinks the body is starving and initiates responses that stop the person losing weight. So if you want to lose weight, combine a sensible diet with plenty of exercise!

BODY TRANSFORMATION

Activity

Mobility exercises/toning and strength

You've now got a comprehensive range of exercises at your disposal that'll help you to further the shaping of your major muscle groups. Warm up first and get stuck right in! Take a 45-second breather between each exercise, otherwise you'll wear yourself out too soon. Concentrate on good posture and technique. And, as always, make sure your technique is steady and controlled.

1. Chair/bench arm dips: 1 set of 15 reps

2. Weighted arm extensions: 1 set of 15 reps

3. Weighted arm curls: 1 set of 15 reps

4. Weighted overhead press: 1 set of 15 reps

5. Weighted side raises: 1 set of 15 reps

6. Weighted front raises: 1 set of 15 reps

7. Weighted bent-over rows: 1 set of 15 reps

8. Alternate leg lunges: 1 set of 20 reps

9. Curl ups: 1 set of 20 reps

10. Bicycles abs: 1 set of 20 reps

11. Hip lifts: 1 set of 20 reps

12. Crossover curls: 1 set of 20 reps (each side)

Every muscle in your body will have had a strenuous workout today so will appreciate being thoroughly stretched. Take your time with each stretch and hold for at least 30 seconds or longer if you've got time.

BODY TRANSFORMATION

Boost your confidence

Most of us have off-days every so often. Here's how to maximise your mood everyday with these confidence-boosting ideas.

Be posture perfect

People who stand tall ooze confidence – so can you! Good posture can make your look a few kilograms lighter as well as relieving tension in your body. Look back at Days 50 to 52 for full advice.

Feel good about yourself

A positive outlook is an attractive quality. A negative self-image, both physically and emotionally, can make you appear anxious, introverted and self-conscious, when in fact, you've probably got lots of great qualities that you can let shine through. Here are a couple of suggestions:

◆ Make a list of all your good qualities. Are you a quick thinker? A good conversationalist? Easy-going? On a bad day, remembering your good points can help to make you more positive.
◆ Try not to be self-critical. For example, instead of thinking, 'I've got big hips', try 'I've got sexy curves'. The more you say it, the more you'll believe it! Feeling good about the way you look helps improve your self-esteem.

Get up 20 minutes early

Don't hit the snooze button – even if it's grey and rainy outside. Use the time to:
◆ Walk (at least part of the way) to work instead of taking the car or public transport. Walking is free, you can tone up, get fresh air and plan your day all at once!
◆ Keep exercising.
◆ Sit down and eat a healthy breakfast. Don't dash out of the house on an empty stomach.

BODY TRANSFORMATION

- Try 10 minutes of meditation or a relaxation exercise to help you chill out and prepare for the day.
- Pamper yourself in the bath or shower.
- Spend more time with your family, even if it's just chatting in bed with your partner or telling stories to your children.
- Do those household chores that you'd usually leave until the weekend.
- Prepare a healthy packed lunch. You'll save money and you'll know exactly what you're eating.
- If you really can't get out of bed, why not wake up to a news or current affairs programme? Research shows that the more active your brain is during your first waking hours, the better it performs during the rest of the day.

TOP TIP

- Enjoy who you are. Look at your fingerprints – you're unique! No one else is exactly like you. The way you laugh and smile and your view on the world is different from everybody else. Acknowledge the whole you and not just your body.

'Let food be thy medicine, thy medicine shall be thy food.'
Hippocrates, Greek physician

Activity

30-minute cardio power walk/slow jog

It's getting tougher now but you know you can rise to the challenge. You're going to push yourself for 30 minutes by fast walking for 50 paces and then jog for 50 paces.

Cool down afterwards with some stretches.

BODY TRANSFORMATION

Back to life

More than 90% of back pain is caused by muscle weakness in the back or abdomen or both. Modern lifestyle habits put a lot of strain on our lower backs. Too much sitting and slouching around, not enough exercise, being overweight and chronic stress can all cause back pain. To avoid it, make sure your posture is good and use exercises to strengthen the muscle groups that sustain your posture.

10 top tips to avoid lower-back pain

1. **Pain is a warning sign** Your body is telling you that you've already caused damage or are about to. If what you're doing hurts, then stop. Don't try to push through the pain.
2. **Regular exercise** Do it regularly and painlessly to help with mobility and strength. Brisk walking, swimming and cycling are all excellent exercises for the lower back.
3. **Warm up** This is crucial before any physical activity, whether it's sports, gardening or DIY. It prepares your body for action and helps to prevent injuries.
4. **Cooling down** Winding down and stretching after exercise are just as important as warming up.
5. **Lift correctly** When you pick something up, no matter how light or heavy, get it as close to your body as you can, keep your back straight and don't twist with it.
6. **Keep on moving** Whether you're at home, at work or in the car, prolonged sitting causes stress on the discs and weakness of the muscles. Get up and move around every now and then, even if it's only for a minute.
7. **Get the right furniture** So-called 'comfortable chairs' don't do your back any good as they force you to slouch and sit awkwardly. Choose a chair that's supportive and allows you to sit up properly with your feet flat on the floor. The right bed is also important. The base should be firm and the mattress soft enough to mould to the contours of your body but firm enough to give you support in the right places. Futons aren't good for most backs. Beds can also be too hard.

BODY TRANSFORMATION

8. **Sleep in a comfortable position** Aim for the foetal position, which is usually the least stressful on your back. Sleeping on your front puts most stress on your back and neck. Choose a pillow that supports your neck.

9. **Use medication for back pain wisely** All drugs have side effects so use them with care. Pain killers such as paracetamol and non-steroidal anti-inflammatory drugs only help to mask the symptoms and do not sort out the problem.

10. **Consult a chiropractor** If you have a long-term problem, whether niggling or disabling, then a chiropractor can probably help. They can usually relieve pain and discomfort, as well as decreasing the likelihood of a recurrence.

Activity

Mobility exercises/toning and strength

You should be standing tall and proud now with your buffed-up bod achieved through sweat and, at times, tears and hard graft! Two sets of every exercise will ensure that you'll be working towards your peak.

1. Chair/bench arm dips: 2 sets of 12 reps
2. Weighted arm extensions: 2 sets of 12 reps
3. Weighted arm curls: 2 sets of 12 reps
4. Weighted overhead press: 2 sets of 12 reps
5. Weighted side raises: 2 sets of 12 reps
6. Weighted front raises: 2 sets of 12 reps
7. Weighted bent-over rows: 2 sets of 12 reps
8. Alternate leg lunges: 2 sets of 12 reps
9. Curl ups: 2 sets of 12 reps
10. Bicycles abs: 2 sets of 12 reps
11. Hip lifts: 2 sets of 12 reps
12. Crossover curls: 2 sets of 12 reps (each side)

As always, don't miss out on the stretches after your workout!

BODY TRANSFORMATION

Body types

For some people, it seems impossible to lose weight. You may be able to blame your body type for this! Your genes determine your body frame and shape and, although you can't completely transform your body type, you can make the most of it by changing your eating habits and exercise. There are three categories of body types: ectomorph, mesomorph and endomorph.

Nobody is 100% one body type. We all have a mixture of body-type characteristics, although one usually dominates.

The ectomorph – key characteristics

- Delicately built and thin
- Flat chest
- Lean and thin
- Lightly muscled and takes longer to gain muscle
- Small shoulders.

The ectomorph has a linear physique with long limbs and a lack of muscle mass. They aren't naturally powerful and will have to work hard to gain muscle and strength.

Famous ectomorphs: Kate Moss, Hilary Swank, Kylie Minogue, Lisa Kudrow, Jude Law, Ed Norton, Leonardo DiCaprio, Tim Henman.

The mesomorph – key characteristics

- Athletic and muscular (gains muscle easily)
- Hourglass shaped (female)
- Rectangular shaped (male)
- Excellent posture
- Gains fat more easily than ectomorphs.

The mesomorph has well-defined muscles and large bones. The torso tends to taper to a relatively narrow and low waist. The bones and muscles of the head are quite prominent.

Famous mesomorphs: Madonna, Cindy Crawford, Jennifer Aniston, Denise Lewis, Sting, Sylvester Stallone, Brad Pitt, Arnold Schwarzenegger.

The endomorph – key characteristics

◆ Soft body with round physique
◆ Underdeveloped muscles
◆ Difficult to lose weight
◆ Gains muscle easily like the mesomorph.

The endomorph's body is round and soft. The arms and legs are shorter with a relatively large abdominal area and a high waist. An endomorph's hands and feet are comparatively small, and the upper arms and thighs are often more developed than the lower parts of the arms or legs.

Famous endomorphs: Roseanne Barr, Oprah Winfrey, Kate Winslet, Sophie Dahl, Lucianno Pavarotti, Orson Welles, Elton John.

Combinations of body types

Nearly all of us fall into mixed categories, such as ecto-mesomorphs or endo-mesomorphs, where we are mostly a mesomoph, but with some ectomorph traits (such as a trim waist) or endomorph traits (such as gaining fat easily).

Regardless of your shape or size, the focus should be on 'healthy' not 'skinny'. You can be a gorgeous healthy endomorph as a result of healthy eating and exercise. No matter which body type you have, you'll harvest the rewards of exercise – a leaner, stronger body. Most importantly, you'll also feel the difference.

Activity

Active rest day

Go for an extra walk today or take the stairs instead of the lift. Stand up every now and then and move around, just to keep your heart pumping and blood flowing.

BODY TRANSFORMATION

Time or timing?

When's the best time to exercise? Whenever suits you best! If you've got the energy and enthusiasm for your workouts, whatever time of day they are, don't change anything. But, if you've been dragging yourself to exercise, here's the low-down on the best time to exercise.

Circadian rhythms

According to research, our bodies follow a daily cycle called circadian rhythms, which regulate your body temperature, metabolism and blood pressure. These rhythms are affected by light and dark and may be re-regulated every day according to factors such as the environment. We're born with our bodies' rhythms, but we reset them every day when our alarm goes off, when we eat and when we exercise. Whenever you change one of these factors, your body reacts as if it has jet lag. It learns to be fittest whenever you usually put it to work. So, if you're off schedule, your stamina may be a bit lower.

Are you a lark or an owl?

If you wake up instantly and cheerfully in the morning but fade early in the evening, you're definitely a lark. If it's hard waking up but you're alive and energetic at night, you're an owl. So, larks prefer morning exercise and owls workout better late in the afternoon or early evening.

When to workout

If your daily routine means you can't exercise at your preferred time, don't despair. Your body can adapt to almost any conditions, given time. Give yourself two to three weeks to adjust if you're switching exercise schedules from morning to afternoon or vice-versa.

BODY TRANSFORMATION

Circadian rhythms affect body temperature. You get the best workout when your body temperature is at its highest and not such a good workout when your temperature is low. For most people, body temperature is at its highest in the late afternoon and at its lowest about one to three hours before you wake in the morning.

Strength is about 5% greater around noon. Aerobic capacity increases by about 4% in the afternoon. Anaerobic performance (rapid intense activities like sprinting) also improves by 5% in the afternoon.

Morning exercisers are more likely to stick with their exercise programmes than people who exercise in the afternoon or evening. This is probably because as the day goes on, it's easy to start making excuses as to why you can't exercise.

Activity

30-minute cardio power walk/slow jog

You're going to increase your jogging paces today by an extra 25 paces. It makes all the difference towards building up your stamina and helping you lose weight. Spend the first 15 minutes of your session power walking at a brisk pace. For the remaining 15 minutes follow a slow, steady jog for 75 paces with 50 paces of power walking.

During stretching, encourage your muscles to stretch that much further by gently pulling a touch more. Breathe and hold. When your muscles have relaxed more, stretch them a little further.

BODY TRANSFORMATION

Your notes

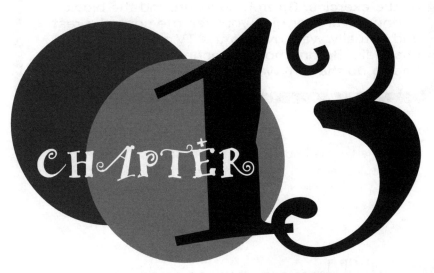

CHAPTER 13

VIM AND VIGOUR

Don't just sit there

Activity

Active rest day

Instead of sitting on the sofa and watching TV, do a little exercise. Stretch, walk around the block during adverts or give your remote control a rest and actually walk over to the TV to change the channels. Before modern technology, some of you had to do that anyway!

'The human body is made up of some four hundred muscles, evolved through centuries of physical activity. Unless these are used, they will deteriorate.'
Eugene Lyman Fisk

TOP TIP 1

◆ Exercising is boring. Breathing is boring, but we do it almost every minute. Find new running routes and notice different things on every run. Stop for a stretch and enjoy the view. Run as close to nature as the elements allow.

VIM AND VIGOUR

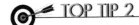

TOP TIP 2

- Sugar-free chewing gum tends to stop you from nibbling bits of food while you're cooking. It might not look very sophisticated when you have guests over, but it could just save you from overeating, and let you enjoy your meal.

MYTH: Water is the only drink I'll ever need.
FACT: Drinking a litre of water every day flushes out and purifies the system. If you drink a glass of water 30 minutes before a meal, it fills up your stomach and makes you eat less. But water doesn't contain vital vitamins and lacks several essential minerals that you get from fruit juice.

MYTH: Drinking alcohol is bad for you.
FACT: Drinking a glass of wine or two is actually good for you. Studies show that those who drink a glass of red wine daily get fewer colds than the average person. Just don't go overboard. More than two glasses can cancel out the benefits. (It's the flavonoids on the grape skin that does the trick!)

VIM AND VIGOUR

203

Run free

Activity ●●●●●●●●●●●●●●●●

30-minute cardio power walk/slow jog

You've reached another level in your fitness and determination now. It's been 12 weeks of hard work, but it's paying great dividends. You're now more than capable of power walking for 10 minutes of your session with a burst of real energy. You're also ready to tackle the follow-on 20 minutes with controlled jogging for 50 paces followed immediately by 100 paces of power walking.

Don't miss out on your stretching afterwards, otherwise you'll feel it tomorrow when you can't walk!

MYTH: Aerobic exercise tends to make you hungry, so it undermines your efforts to lose weight.
FACT: Aerobic exercise, such as jogging or brisk walking, may increase your appetite – but only, it seems, if you need extra calories. Studies suggest that lean individuals do get hungrier after such exercise, which helps stop them getting too thin. By contrast, working out doesn't seem to boost appetite in people who are overweight, so exercise should help them slim down.

'Dieting is like a plane journey. You have to get off at some stage!'
Anonymous

TOP TIP 1

- Make sure your plate is half veggies and/or fruit at both lunch and dinner.

 TOP TIP 2

- Take the stairs whenever you can. If you've got a meeting on the 14th floor, get out of the lift a few floors early and use the stairs.

MYTH: Women who exercise will have trouble delivering babies.

FACT: Years ago, you'd be unlikely to find a pregnant woman at the gym or health club. Doctors then were afraid that exercise would lead to birth defects or encourage a miscarriage. Today, it's a different ball game altogether. More and more women are taking up exercise. And if you're pregnant, the right exercise, for example, pregnancy yoga, can be good for your baby and will make childbirth easy. Not only is moderate exercise safe for your baby, but it also has tremendous benefits for mum. Compared to unfit pregnant women, pregnant women who exercise regularly tend to have fewer aches and pains, better self-esteem, and more energy and stamina, especially in the third trimester. Regular exercisers also have more confidence – and perhaps strength – during labour and they seem to tolerate pain better.

VIM AND VIGOUR

Keep the technique

Activity

Mobility exercises/toning and strength

Concentrate on your posture and make sure you keep your stomach muscles drawn in during these exercises. Constantly be aware of your technique and control to get the most out of these exercises. You're upping your reps today to 15!

1. Chair/bench arm dips: 2 sets of 15 reps

2. Weighted arm extensions: 2 sets of 15 reps

3. Weighted arm curls: 2 sets of 15 reps

4. Weighted overhead press: 2 sets of 15 reps

5. Weighted side raises: 2 sets of 15 reps

6. Weighted front raises: 2 sets of 15 reps

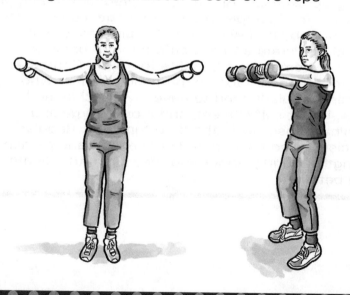

7. Weighted bent-over rows: 2 sets of 15 reps

8. Chair leg squats: 2 sets of 15 reps

9. Alternate leg lunges: 2 sets of 15 reps

10. Curl ups: 2 sets of 15 reps

11. Bicycles abs: 2 sets of 15 reps

12. Hip lifts: 2 sets of 15 reps

13. Crossover curls: 2 sets of 15 reps

Stretch, stretch, stretch and more stretching afterwards!

'Exercise isn't a necessary evil. It's a necessary good.' Cornel Chin

TOP TIP 1

◆ See what you eat. Put your food on a plate or in a bowl instead of eating out of the jar or bag.

TOP TIP 2

◆ Why not set up a community group to form walking clubs, build walking trails, start exercise classes and organise special events to promote physical activity?

MYTH: Obesity is genetic.
FACT: Only one percent of obese people can blame their parents. The obesity epidemic is down to sedentary lifestyles combined with energy-rich and fat-laden diets.

VIM AND VIGOUR

Step up your pace

Activity

Cardio power walk/slow jog

Spend the first 10 minutes of your session power walking at a brisk pace. During the following 20 minutes go for a slow, steady jog for 50 paces followed immediately by 50 paces of power walking.

Treat yourself to some relaxation time. During your stretches, feel all of the tension being released from your body. Clear your mind and think only positive, happy thoughts.

TOP TIP 1

◆ Make sure your workout is convenient. Schedule it for a time of day when you usually feel the most energetic. Have your gear packed and ready to go by the door or in the car.

TOP TIP 2

- Keep seven bags of your favourite frozen vegetables to hand. Mix any combination, microwave and top with your favourite low-fat dressing. Enjoy three to four cups a day. This makes a great quick dinner!

TOP TIP 3

- Never be depressed about your weight. Stress keeps you fat – it can slow down your metabolism to preserve energy – so look on the brighter side of things!

'The answer to the perfect body isn't found in a tub of ice cream or a box of tricks.' Cornel Chin

MYTH: People are overweight because they have slow metabolisms.
FACT: Unfortunately, a slow metabolism is no excuse for being overweight. In fact, recent studies have shown that fat people have faster metabolisms and burn off more energy than slimmer people simply to keep their bodies going. There are other factors that may cause metabolic problems, such as heredity and hormones, for example thyroid and insulin imbalances – but these cases are rare!

VIM AND VIGOUR

Are you keeping up? Do you need some help? If you've not already subscribed, why not try the daily text messaging service for extra encouragement and support.
Just text 'Body Idol 81' to 80881 now.

Each set of messages costs £1.50. Please see page xiv for full terms and conditions.

Say no to lazy bones

Active rest day

Think of different ways to keep your body moving today.

TOP TIP 1

◆ Don't let cold weather or rain keep you on the sofa. You can still find activities to do like exercising indoors or joining a sports league. Or get a head start on your spring cleaning by choosing active indoor chores like window cleaning or reorganising cupboards.

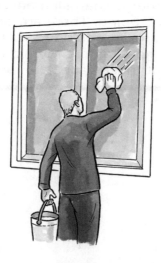

TOP TIP 2

- ◆ When out walking, bring along the dog or strap your child into a jogging stroller or pushchair. If they count on you for their daily dose of fresh air, you'll have an added reason to get out there!

TOP TIP 3

- ◆ Make decisions about what you're going to eat. Weight management is all about moderation and making healthy decisions.

MYTH: When you get older, your muscles turn into fat.

FACT: Muscle and fat are two different types of body tissue. Muscle can't be converted into fat or vice versa. This myth stems from the number of die-hard exercise fanatics who stop training once they're older or retired. Once they retire, they tend to add fat and lose muscle because they're used to eating well and they carry on doing so even when they don't burn calories through exercise anymore. So, their muscles shrink and they add body fat, making it seem as if they somehow converted their muscles into fat.

VIM AND VIGOUR

Shape that body

Activity

Mobility exercises/toning and strength

This is a big giant leap forward in your toning and strength work today as you'll add in an extra set of every exercise after you've warmed up. It's essential that you have a 45-second rest between each exercise so you can recuperate properly.

1. Chair/bench arm dips: 3 sets of 12 reps

2. Weighted arm extensions: 3 sets of 12 reps

3. Weighted arm curls: 3 sets of 12 reps

4. Weighted overhead press: 3 sets of 12 reps

5. Weighted side raises: 3 sets of 12 reps

6. Weighted front raises: 3 sets of 12 reps

7. Weighted bent-over rows: 3 sets of 12 reps

8. Chair leg squats: 3 sets of 12 reps

9. Alternate leg lunges: 3 sets of 12 reps

10. Curl ups: 3 sets of 12 reps

11. Bicycles abs: 3 sets of 12 reps

12. Hip lifts: 3 sets of 12 reps

13. Crossover curls: 3 sets of 12 reps (each side)

Work, play and rest – finish off by doing some stretching!

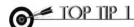

TOP TIP 1

◆ Wouldn't it be easier to eat something if it was right in front of you? An easy way to make fruit and vegetables more accessible is to make sure you buy them. Makes sense, right? So when you go food shopping, hit the fruit and veg section first. Then keep bowls of fruit on the kitchen table and worktop. Now that you've bought them, eat them!

TOP TIP 2

◆ Make a date...to exercise. You're more likely to carry on exercising if you enjoy it. The health benefits and calories burned are a bonus! Preparation plus the right attitude equals for achievement. Make regular exercise a habit and you're more likely to stick with it. At 4 pm, you shouldn't be thinking, 'Shall I exercise tonight?' because it sets you up to refuse. Instead, think, 'What exercise shall I do this tonight?'

MYTH: Dieting makes me mentally sharper and more alert.
FACT: Dieting dulls the mind. Studies have shown there's a link between dieting and mental performance. The reduction in working memory capacity occurs because slimmers' brains are so preoccupied with dieting that other brain processes don't get a look in!

VIM AND VIGOUR

Put a spring in your step

Activity Cardio power walk/slow jog

You're really on your way now to a super sleek, sexier body. It's not all about the look though. Think about what's going on inside you. A lower heart rate, more efficient lungs, raised metabolic rate and an all-round healthier body. These are just a few of the positive effects of exercise. To springboard you on to greater improvement, you're going to complete the first five minutes of your session walking at a rapid, but well-controlled pace. You'll then do the remaining 25 minutes combining a steady jog for 50 paces with 100 paces of power walking.

Now target those hard-worked leg muscles with some well-earned stretches.

'True enjoyment comes from activity of the mind and exercise of the body; the two are ever united.' Alexander von Humboldt, explorer and naturalist

TOP TIP 1

♦ Forgo the lift in favour of the stairs. Climb stairs as a workout in itself. Stand on the bottom step and do backward lunges onto the landing. Use the second step to do triceps dips.

VIM AND VIGOUR

214

TOP TIP 2

♦ Baked potatoes, corn on the cob, bread. You love to cover them with butter, right? And if you're not careful – and it's easily done – you don't realise how much you actually use. If you must use butter and margarine, use them sparingly. Even better, switch to reduced-fat margarine on your bread, bagels and jacket potatoes.

TOP TIP 3

♦ Pick one place at home and one at work as a place to eat. Be sure you're sitting down as this focuses your attention more directly on eating. Don't eat anywhere else. By eating in the same place every day, you identify and associate that place with eating. Enjoy your food by eating slowly.

MYTH: Skipping breakfast means one less meal a day resulting in fewer calories.
FACT: Breakfast is the most important meal and eating it can help you to lose weight. The body's internal chemistry is at its most active first thing in the morning, so anything eaten then will be used to the maximum. By skipping breakfast, you may end up eating more because you feel hungrier during the day.

VIM AND VIGOUR

Your notes

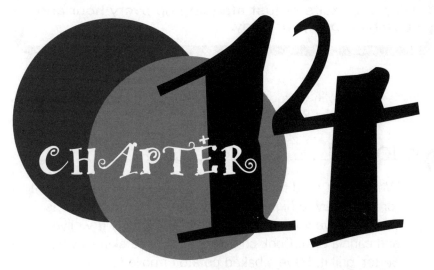

CHAPTER 14

THOSE UNFIT DAYS
ARE LONG GONE

Creative activity

Activity ●●●●●●●●●●●●●●
Active rest day

Try to be more active today by working in the garden, walking the dog, walking to the shops, using the stairs or just standing up every hour and stretching out your body.

'Preserving health by too severe a rule is a worrisome malady.'
François La Rochefoucauld, French classical author

⦿ ← TOP TIP 1

◆ What about fried foods? They taste great, but aren't great for you. They're high in fat. Here are a few suggestions that will save your arteries. Use oils sparingly (try olive and canola oils). Cook chicken without the skin – even better, grill it. Have a baked potato or boiled potatoes instead of chips.

⦿ ← TOP TIP 2

◆ Exercise shouldn't be a temporary fad. It should be for life.

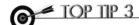

TOP TIP 3

- Forget about big, bulky workout equipment. Tone your arms with basic strengthening exercises using light weights or household items such as tin cans. Do standing push ups against a wall.

MYTH: Women have the same physical capabilities as men.
FACT: Apart from the obvious, the main physical differences between the sexes are that men have approximately 50% more muscle mass than women as well as greater bone mass. The female body accumulates approximately 10% more body fat than the man. The size of an average man's heart is 25% larger than the average woman's, and the lung capacity in men is about 27% greater than in women.

MYTH: If a woman lifts weights, she'll get 'bulky'.
FACT: Very few women have enough testosterone that can lead to big size increases. As muscle is denser than fat, if you replace one kilo of fat on a body part with one kilo of muscle, the body part will be much smaller and denser. Women who seem 'bulky' are simply carrying around too much body fat.

THOSE UNFIT DAYS ARE LONG GONE

Jog for joy

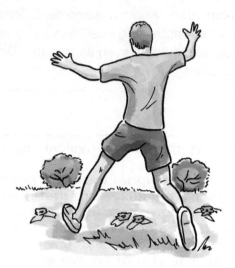

Activity

Cardio power walk/slow jog

Get your training shoes on and get out there! It's the same 30 minutes, but with a slight change in the mix. You'll spend five minutes of your session walking quickly. Then for 25 minutes, alternate 75 paces of jogging with 100 paces of fast walking.

Lengthen out your body now with a good stretch routine.

TOP TIP 1

♦ Why do we eat snacks? They taste great, they're easy and they satisfy our sweet and salt cravings. And, let's face it, crunchy food is fun. So why not make your own snacks by packing healthy, quick-and-easy-to-grab foods such as little bags or containers of ready-to-eat vegetables (e.g. celery sticks, cucumber wedges and cherry tomatoes) and fruit. Or make healthier choices on snacks that are bought from the shop, like rice cakes. Keep them with you in your bag, office, car and home.

TOP TIP 2

♦ Too cramped, too crowded or too crazed? If your home environment isn't fit for a good workout, head out the door in search of greener pastures.

MYTH: If it tastes good, it must be bad.
FACT: Not exactly a myth, but it's a thought that often crosses your mind and makes you smile when you're eating something tasty. The opposite is true too – when you eat something awful, you tend to think it must be good for you, although this isn't always the case either!

THOSE UNFIT DAYS ARE LONG GONE

Challenge your muscles

Activity

Mobility exercises/toning and strength

Warm up first. Now, how about increasing your reps by three today? Your mantra when doing these exercises is 'Tone, tone and more tone!'

1. Chair/bench arm dips: 3 sets of 15 reps

2. Weighted arm extensions: 3 sets of 15 reps

3. Weighted arm curls: 3 sets of 15 reps

4. Weighted overhead press: 3 sets of 15 reps

5. Weighted side raises: 3 sets of 15 reps

6. Weighted front raises: 3 sets of 15 reps

7. Weighted bent-over rows: 3 sets of 15 reps

8. Chair leg squats: 3 sets of 15 reps

9. Alternate leg lunges: 3 sets of 15 reps

10. Curl ups: 3 sets of 15 reps

11. Bicycles abs: 3 sets of 15 reps

12. Hip lifts: 3 sets of 15 reps

13. Crossover curls: 3 sets of 15 reps (each side)

Make the effort to stretch a bit longer today. Your body needs it!

THOSE UNFIT DAYS ARE LONG GONE

'If the beginning is good, the end must be perfect.'
Burmese proverb

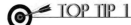 TOP TIP 1

- ◆ To make packed lunches more interesting, opt for healthy fillings such as ham, beef, turkey, skinless chicken, canned sardines, salmon, hard-boiled egg, Edam, mozzarella and low-fat cream cheese.

TOP TIP 2

- ◆ If you've tried to get fit in the past but didn't succeed, don't throw in the towel. Learn from your mistakes. Re-evaluate what went wrong and try again.

MYTH: There's so little of it, it can't be fattening!
FACT: This myth is popular when it comes to foods like spare ribs, cheesecake or any other calorie-rich food that you think 'just a little of' won't make a calorie-iota of difference to your diet. Although portion size is a very important consideration when dieting, you have to remember that what's in the portion, as well as how it's prepared, also makes a difference. Just because it's a small amount, doesn't mean it doesn't count. Spare ribs are still fatty and high in calories and if they're drenched in a rich sauce you might want to steer yourself over to the salad bar instead. Also bear in mind that 'just a sliver' of cheesecake or a 'mouthful' of chocolate-coated nuts could cost you 500 calories. Another trap is that 'just a little' can lead to 'just a little bit more'. Again, you need to keep counting those calories to keep aware of exactly what you're eating.

THOSE UNFIT DAYS ARE LONG GONE

223

Run for fun

Activity **Cardio power walk/slow jog**

Spend the first five minutes of your session power walking at a brisk pace. Then alternate the remaining 25 minutes between a slow, steady jog for 75 paces and 75 paces of power walking.

Keep on stretching!

'Believing you're immune to being fit and healthy is both ignorant and idle.' Cornel Chin

MYTH: Bananas, carrots and tomatoes will make you gain weight.

FACT: The idea behind this one is that bananas, carrots and tomatoes are high in sugar and calories compared to broccoli and other fruit and vegetables. Sounds like something out of a 60s diet book, doesn't it? Well, it probably was. And while most fad diet ideas come and go before you can say 'that's ridiculous', this is one that's hung around. When it comes down to it, it's really a question of relativity: Arnold Schwarzenegger probably feels big until he stands next to a basketball player, and a banana is sugary until you put it next to a chocolate bar. Perhaps carrots and tomatoes have 5–10 more calories than a portion of broccoli, but try them against a bag of crisps or a handful of chocolate buttons!

TOP TIP 1

- Don't tell yourself, 'It's okay, it's the holidays.' That opens the door to six weeks of splurging and added kilos with every party, biscuit and drink.

TOP TIP 2

- Keeping a note in your fitness notebook to show improvements will help you see how well you're doing and can help you set new goals. If you feel like you've been doing the same thing for ages, set a new challenge and track your progress. Having some workout 'homework' could help you become more diligent.

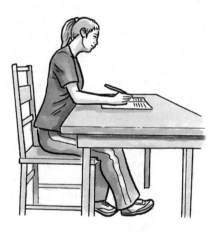

THOSE UNFIT DAYS ARE LONG GONE

Get mean with the clean

Activity

Active rest day

How clean is your house? Today, invest some time and effort in sprucing up your pad. It will be sparklingly clean with the added benefit of burning off several hundred calories.

'A good man and health is a woman's best wealth.'
English proverb

MYTH: Grapefruit burns fat.
FACT: There always seems to be some magical food that's going to make you burn fat. Grapefruit is a pretty popular one, but there are also claims that cabbage soup, yoghurt and certain herbs can make you lose weight by burning fat. Interestingly, new research suggests that eating grapefruit can actually help people to lose weight – but not because it burns fat. A 12-week study of obese patients showed that those who ate fresh grapefruit or drank grapefruit juice every day lost an average 1.4 kilos more than those who didn't eat grapefruit. Researchers believe something in grapefruit may turn off the desire to eat more food. Some foods high in caffeine, as well as certain herbs and spices, may increase metabolism, but that doesn't make you lose weight. Again, it's the calories that count, so count those calories.

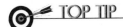 TOP TIP

- Walk around the shopping centre three times before you start shopping – your health and your purse will love you for it!

MYTH: While light exercise does yield some benefits, it's not nearly as beneficial as strenuous exercise.

FACT: Strenuous workouts do improve aerobic capacity far more than light or moderate workouts do. While that may improve althletic performance, it does not necessarily translate into a great health advantage. Experts state that the death rates from coronary heart disease, cancer and all causes combined are much lower in moderate exercisers than in non exercisers; but they're only a little lower in heavy exercisers than in moderate exercisers. The same holds true for the risk of developing type II diabetes, by far the most common kind. In addition, non strenuous exercise seems to reduce stress, anxiety and blood pressure as effectively as strenuous exercise does. And moderate exercise like walking can do just as much to control weight as vigorous exercise like jogging, since the number of calories burned depends on how much ground you cover, not how fast you cover it. In fact, moderate exercise is potentially more effective than vigorous for most people, since they can walk much further than they can run.

THOSE UNFIT DAYS ARE LONG GONE

Every stride counts

Activity Cardio power walk/slow jog

Great work – you're at a high level of fitness and in great condition now. Make the effort to walk and jog as best as you can. Daily progression is the key here – you've challenged your body to be able to improve upon it. If you don't challenge it, it will only exert itself enough for the task in hand. Work hard and make every stride count. It's five minutes fast walking today and 25 minutes steady jogging for 75 paces alternated with 50 paces of power walking.

Hold and control all of your stretches for at least 45 seconds.

'The sickness of the body may prove the health of the soul.'
Chinese proverb

 TOP TIP 1

- ◆ Try two weeks without sweets. It's amazing how your cravings vanish.

THOSE UNFIT DAYS ARE LONG GONE

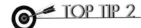

TOP TIP 2

♦ Natural athletic ability is not a prerequisite to physical activity. Simply go and do what comes easiest and naturally, but keep on moving!

MYTH: Processed foods are not as nutritious as fresh foods.

FACT: Many processed foods are just as nutritious or in some cases even more nutritious than fresh foods depending on how they're processed. Frozen vegetables are usually processed within hours of harvest. There's little nutrient loss in the freezing process so frozen vegetables keep their high vitamin and mineral content. By contrast, fresh vegetables are picked and transported to market. It can take days or even weeks before they reach the dinner table and vitamins are graduallly lost over time no matter how carefully the vegetables are transported and stored. Some processed foods, such as breads and breakfast cereals, have vitamins and minerals added for extra nutrition. The growing interest in health and nutrition has spurred on the production of a whole new range of foods with added health and nutritional benefits, such as fat spreads with added fibre to lower cholesterol. Processing can also make some nutrients more available. For example, removing phytic acid from grain foods by removing the bran helps to improve the absorption of iron. Processing tomatoes into a tomato paste or sauce increases the amount of lycopene (an antioxidant) available to the body.

THOSE UNFIT DAYS ARE LONG GONE

Sports fan

Activity

Active rest day

Have you ever thought about learning a new sport or returning to an old sport that you haven't played for donkey's years? Well, today is the day. Grab that old tennis racket or hockey stick and brush off the cobwebs – now go and round up your friends and shout 'Anyone for tennis!' or 'Jolly hockey sticks!' Why not try one of the following:

- Swimming
- Badminton
- Netall
- Squash
- Dance
- Horse riding
- Canoeing
- Aerobics
- Golf
- Orienteering
- Cycling
- Kickboxing
- Rowing

The list is endless...

'Who is more busy than he that has least to do?' Chinese proverb

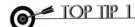

TOP TIP 1

♦ Eat your evening meal in the kitchen or dining room sitting down at your table.

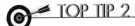

TOP TIP 2

♦ Working out should be a challenge, but it definitely shouldn't be painful. If you find yourself running straight for the ice packs and aspirin after working out, you're probably doing something wrong. Before you convince yourself you've got a wonderful excuse to give up, try evaluating your exercise programme.

MYTH: Overweight people are unlikely to benefit much from exercise.
FACT: Studies show that obese people who take part in regular exercise programmes have a lower risk of all-cause mortality than sedentary individuals, regardless of weight. Both men and women of all sizes and fitness levels can improve their health with modest increases in activity.

THOSE UNFIT DAYS ARE LONG GONE

Your notes

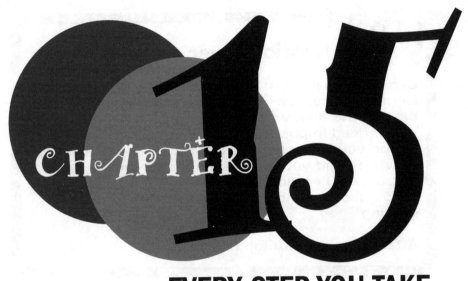

CHAPTER 15

EVERY STEP YOU TAKE

Are you keeping up? Do you need some help? If you've not already subscribed, why not try the daily text messaging service for extra encouragement and support.
Just text 'Body Idol 91' to 80881 now.

Each set of messages costs £1.50. Please see page xiv for full terms and conditions.

Mission possible

Activity
Cardio power walk/slow jog

Can you believe that you're actually jogging for this length of time? It's hard to imagine if you reflect back to the time when you thought the impossible was indeed impossible. Give yourself a great big pat on your back (you've got the flexibility to reach now!). Spend your first five minutes walking at a fast pace. Then do 25 minutes of steady jogging for 50 paces combined with 50 paces of power walking.

Afterwards, it's stretch out time!

'By doing nothing we learn to do ill.' Japanese proverb

 TOP TIP 1

♦ Eat without doing something else at the same time. No reading, watching TV or sitting at your computer. You can easily lose track of how much you're eating.

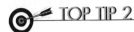

TOP TIP 2

- Didn't feel like working out today? When you feel the temptations to skip your workouts or hear that little voice saying 'I can start again next month', remind yourself of the reasons that you want to exercise. Write down on an index card the main reasons why you should exercise. Keep this in a prominent place… maybe in your office or wherever you spend a great deal of time.

MYTH: The health and fitness benefits of mind–body exercise like tai chi and yoga are questionable.
FACT: In fact, research showing the benefits of these exercises continues to grow. Tai chi, for example, has been shown to help treat lower-back pain and fibromyalgia. Improved flexibility, balance, co-ordination, posture, strength and stress management are just some of the potential results of mind–body exercises.

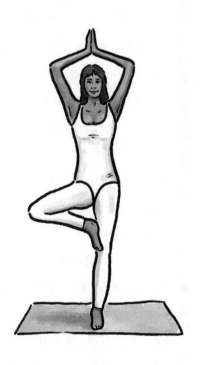

EVERY STEP YOU TAKE

Bye, bye wobbly bits

Activity

Mobility exercises/toning and strength

All 13 exercises are now three sets of 18 reps, which is great! Your body's showing real signs of improvement, which should make you feel stronger and more confident. Remain focused on each exercise, each repetition and each set. Do each rep a little slower and focus on resisting the movement upwards and downwards.

1. Chair/bench arm dips: 3 sets of 18 reps

2. Weighted arm extensions: 3 sets of 18 reps

3. Weighted arm curls: 3 sets of 18 reps

4. Weighted overhead press: 3 sets of 18 reps

5. Weighted side raises: 3 sets of 18 reps

6. Weighted front raises: 3 sets of 18 reps

7. Weighted bent-over rows: 3 sets of 18 reps

8. Chair leg squats: 3 sets of 18 reps

9. Alternate leg lunges: 3 sets of 18 reps

10. Curl ups: 3 sets of 18 reps

11. Bicycles abs: 3 sets of 18 reps

12. Hip lifts: 3 sets of 18 reps

13. Crossover curls: 3 sets of 18 reps (each side)

Now your muscles have been stimulated beyond their normal level, make sure you provide them with lots of stretching.

EVERY STEP YOU TAKE

'Sloth, like rust, consumes faster than labour wears.'
Arabic proverb

TOP TIP 1

♦ Fat-free isn't always your best bet and doesn't mean low in calories. Research has found that none of the alpha- or beta-carotene that fights cancer and heart disease is absorbed from salads with fat-free dressing. Only slightly more is absorbed with reduced-fat dressing. The most is absorbed with full-fat dressing. But remember to use dressing in moderate amounts and have it on the side.

TOP TIP 2

♦ If you've been ill and haven't exercised in weeks, don't think, 'What's the use?' Setbacks will happen... so just accept them. We all have setbacks, but people who are successful on their fitness programmes jump right back on track as soon as they can. Don't let setbacks get you down. Be determined and get right back to your routine.

MYTH: Water fitness programmes are primarily for older people or people with injuries.
FACT: Recent research has shown that water fitness programmes (aka aqua workouts) can be highly challenging and effective both for improving fitness and losing weight. Even top athletes integrate water fitness workouts into their training programmes. It's a great alternative to other methods of exercising.

EVERY STEP YOU TAKE

Silent running

Activity

Cardio power walk/slow jog

Pump your arms to get them up above the level of your heart. You should be feeling more relaxed about using your arms and less worried about how you look doing it by now. Who cares how it looks? Your aim is to enjoy yourself and reap the benefits for your body. You've nearly finished your programme so make the most of it. Today, it's five minutes of power walking followed by 25 minutes of jogging for 75 paces combined with 50 paces of power walking.

To keep your legs long and lean and free from tightness, you know it's wise to finish with a little stretching.

TOP TIP 1

♦ Eat breakfast, lunch and dinner. If you miss one of these meals, there's a real risk that you'll struggle with late-night eating and binging.

TOP TIP 2

♦ If you're starving by 4pm and have no alternative but the office vending machine, reach for the fruit or drink water. Sometimes when you feel hungry, what you're actually feeling is dehydrated.

TOP TIP 3

♦ If you're not really a fitness buff, develop the mindset that you're a fitness buff. See yourself as one… and you can become one! Of course it takes action too. Keep a regular exercise schedule and make fitness and healthy eating a priority in your life.

MYTH: Fish oil is fattening.
FACT: Fish oil is high in many beneficial nutrients and studies reveal that heart patients who consumed 1 gram of fish oil a day were 45% less likely to die of unexpected, heart related problems.

EVERY STEP YOU TAKE

Keep on movin'

Activity
Active rest day

You should have formed some great habits and learned to build more activity into your lifestyle in general. Whether at home, at work or on holiday, you know you can keep on moving. These are the tools to becoming a lean, mean, fat-burning machine!

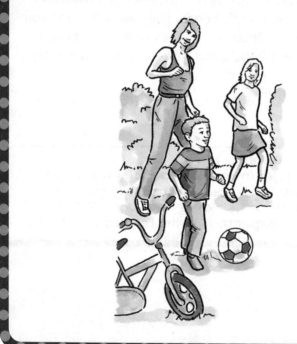

'He who makes no mistakes, makes nothing.' Anonymous

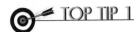

TOP TIP 1

- Overeating isn't the result of exercise. Vigorous exercise won't stimulate you to overeat. It's just the opposite – exercise at any level helps curb your appetite immediately following your workout.

TOP TIP 2

- Goals keep you going. As human beings we're wired for goals. Without goals, you'll simply flounder around with no purpose or direction.

MYTH: Liquids don't really count.

FACT: This tall tale is more of a psychological trick than anything else. If you get your meals in liquid form or drink lots of orange juice, fizzy drinks, lattes and milk, it feels like you're not really eating. When you're counting calories, it's easier to dismiss a glass of orange juice than a sandwich. But the calories don't know whether you're chewing them or not! Water is the only truly calorie-free drink that exists and it's good for you, so drink up. Black tea and black coffee are also very low in calories, but as soon as you start adding sugar, milk and cappuccino foam, they quickly become cupfuls of calories. For example, Vanilla Cream Frappuccino can contain around 700 calories! A skimmed milk Iced Café Latte can still contain 110 calories. Juice, milk and fizzy drinks also have a fair few calories. If you're trying to lose weight, don't forget to count what you slurp, as well as what you munch.

EVERY STEP YOU TAKE

Running wild

Activity
Cardio power walk/slow jog

It's only a few more days to go until you've fulfilled your challenge of jogging for 30 minutes. Really focus on keeping your arms and legs in time with each other. Get the best workout you can in the time you've got. It's five minutes of fast walking first, then 25 minutes of jogging for 100 paces followed by 50 paces of fast walking.

Never skip your stretches, as you're more likely to end up sore and stiff tomorrow.

TOP TIP 1

- ◆ Eat more fruit. If you get enough fruit in your diet, the chances are that you won't have a raging sweet tooth.

TOP TIP 2

- ◆ Stock up on dried fruit. Dried fruit is low in fat and high in fibre. A good handful also counts as one of your fruit servings for the day.

⌖ TOP TIP 3

◆ Accept who you are as you are right now while preparing
and planning for change and growth in the future. At 20
you're a very different person from when you were 12
and you'll be different at 40 and at 60. Your view of the
world will grow and change with your life experiences
and the knowledge you acquire along the way. Remind
yourself how wonderful you are!

MYTH: Strength training builds muscle and bone
but doesn't do a thing for the heart.
FACT: Strength training plus aerobic exercise may
be the ideal exercise regime not only for the
waistline but also for the heart. One analysis of 11
clinical trials found that strength training can
reduce levels of LDL cholesterol (the artery-
clogging kind), although it has little effect on HDL
cholesterol, the artery-clearing kind. Aerobic
exercise has a complimentary benefit – it improves
HDL but does little for LDL. Some studies also
suggest that strength training, like aerobic
exercise, may help reduce blood pressure. One
final benefit: by fortifying the muscles, strength
training reduces the likelihood that sudden or
unaccustomed exertion, such as moving furniture
or shovelling snow, will trigger a heart attack.

EVERY STEP YOU TAKE

Take it to the max

Activity

Mobility exercises/toning and strength

You've now reached your maximum number of reps and sets on all of these exercises. This is a fantastic achievement. Just check and double check that your overall posture and positions are correct and that your pace is strict. Don't forget – quality counts as much as quantity! Always make sure you do some warming up first.

1. Chair/bench arm dips: 3 sets of 18 reps

2. Weighted arm extensions: 3 sets of 20 reps

3. Weighted arm curls: 3 sets of 20 reps

4. Weighted overhead press: 3 sets of 20 reps

5. Weighted side raises: 3 sets of 20 reps

6. Weighted front raises: 3 sets of 20 reps

7. Weighted bent-over rows: 3 sets of 20 reps

8. Chair leg squats: 3 sets of 20 reps

9. Alternate leg lunges: 3 sets of 20 reps

10. Curl ups: 3 sets of 20 reps

11. Bicycles abs: 3 sets of 20 reps

12. Hip lifts: 3 sets of 20 reps

13. Crossover curls: 3 sets of 20 reps (each side)

Stretching is equally as important as your aerobic and toning work, so don't give up on it.

'He that eats till he is sick must fast till he is well.' English proverb

TOP TIP 1

♦ Nuts are healthy but high in calories. Use them as a garnish instead of a snack.

TOP TIP 2

♦ Recognise that it will be easy to exercise on some days, while on others you'll have to struggle through the workout. This has to do with a lot of factors, including mood, hormones, the glass of wine you had last night, etc. Take the pressure off by understanding the fluctuations. And exercise anyway!

MYTH: It's impossible to over exercise.
FACT: The most common injuries from any form of exercise are from overdoing it. Studies show that over exercise actually weakens your immune system, making you more prone to colds, flu and serious medical problems.

EVERY STEP YOU TAKE

Marathon, here I come!

Activity — Cardio power walk/slow jog

This is a giant leap forward as you're nearing the end of your 100-day programme. You're so nearly there! Keep on pushing hard today. Get your heart pumping and your body burning off fat. Spend the first five minutes of your session power walking at a brisk pace. You'll spend the rest of the 25 minutes alternating between a steady jog for 120 paces and 75 paces of power walking.

Familiarity can lead to boredom, so try mixing up your stretches a bit more.

'Greedy eaters dig their graves with their teeth.'
Greek proverb

TOP TIP

◆ How's this for motivation... a pair of size 10 Levis hanging at the back of your wardrobe. You'll not only want to wear those jeans but you want them falling off!

MYTH: Never drink liquids while exercising.
FACT: It was once thought that drinking liquids would bloat the body and affect performance. But the opposite is true. Boxers, dancers, football players and long-distance runners may lose as much as two kilos while performing – most of it water.

Not drinking water while exercising and during hot, humid weather makes an exerciser susceptible to heat cramps, heat exhaustion or the more serious and sometimes fatal heat stroke. Dehydration causes fatigue, which makes you more vulnerable to injury. To improve exercise performance, don't wait until you're thirsty before you drink. By that time, you may already be dehydrated. Instead, drink water before, during and after exercising. Drink about eight fluid ounces of water every 20 minutes while exercising.

MYTH: When you start losing weight, the first few kilos you lose are water. That means water has weight and you have to drink less water if you want to keep your weight down.
FACT: The first sentence is true. The second is false. Drink lots of water – you need it. Yes, losing water causes weight loss at first, but denying yourself water doesn't cause more weight loss in the future, and drinking more water rarely causes weight gain.

EVERY STEP YOU TAKE

Mind gym

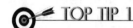

Active rest day

- For a change, train your brain – put your feet up and whip out your inspirational fitness magazines.

- Read articles on how other likeminded people have succeeded. Soon enough you'll be writing your own fitness biography!

'Success is when you can look beyond food... and look down and see your feet.' Cornel Chin

TOP TIP 1

- The longer you're able to stick with your exercise programme, the more likely you are to make permanent lifestyle changes that lead to lasting success!

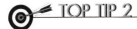

TOP TIP 2

♦ Every day you stay on your weight-loss diet brings you closer to your goal weight.

TOP TIP 3

♦ Remember, sticking with an exercise programme and a healthy diet is more than just motivation. It takes discipline, patience and a constant, daily commitment to your goals. There aren't any shortcuts when it comes to health and fitness but, once you make it a part of your life, you won't regret it!
Repeat: 'I'm learning a way to live, not just a way to diet.'

MYTH: Exercise has to be strenuous to be beneficial.
FACT: You don't have to push yourself to extremes to get the benefits of exercise. In fact, if you exercise excessively, you run the risk of overtraining. Alternate hard workout days with easier ones. And don't forget to rest. If you need to recuperate from difficult workouts, take two to three days off or do less intense exercise – for example, walk instead of jog or run – this will really give your body a chance to recover.

EVERY STEP YOU TAKE

The proof is in the pudding

Activity Cardio power walk/slow jog

- I'd hate this to sound like the end, but it's just the end of one chapter in your life and the beginning of much more success to come. You must be itching to know just how well you've really done, so get out your tape measure, scales, pen and exercise mat. Then, refer to the section on fitness evaluation in Appendix 2 and start testing again. Record your results and tot up your scores!

- Give yourself a pat on the back for coming this far – it's such an achievement. Bask in the knowledge that you're fitter and healthier and possess greater willpower to overcome whatever life throws at you. Stride out for a better life. Spend the first five minutes of your session power walking at a brisk pace. It's then jogging all the way to the finishing line for the final 25 minutes.

- Get comfy on the floor and spend time looking back on your achievements during the last 100 days as you spend time stretching out your body.

You now have the information that you need to succeed in achieving a new life and the bone-idle days are forgotten and never to return – ever.

If you miss a day or two of your workout plan, don't worry. Just pick up where you left off. At the end of this programme you should still feel fitter, firmer and, above all, confident about staying that way forever. You'll never look back.

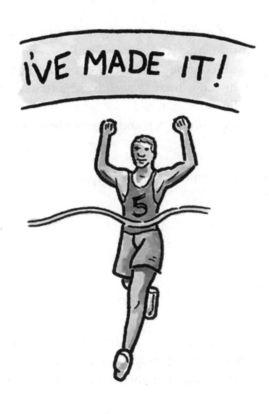

Where do I go from here?

You may be wondering, 'Where do I go from here?' Your new-found vitality and fitness will spur you on to do more adventurous activities:

♦ Why not take part in a sponsored run? Not only will it increase your motivation, but you'll be raising money for a good cause.

♦ You might find that watching top sports live or on television will ignite your passion to take up a new sport or improve an existing one.

♦ Learning a form of martial arts is a dynamic way of promoting self-discipline and improving your fitness level.

♦ Of course, you can continue with your current programme, making alterations to your time, distance, weights and number of repetitions as the exercises become easier.

♦ The world is now your oyster, and there's plenty out there for the taking!

Remember the golden rules that have helped you to achieve a healthy, shapely body:

1. Exercise.
2. Eat healthily.
3. Get adequate rest.
4. Get plenty of fresh air.
5. Accept yourself.

Adopt a positive and peaceful approach to yourself, focus on what you know are good points rather than what you think might be your worst, and be happy. These are the ingredients for your continued success!

Why not try another title in the **GET A LIFE!** series?

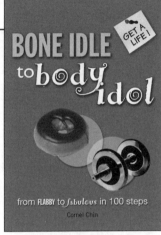

BONE IDLE to BODY IDOL

0-340-90799-1

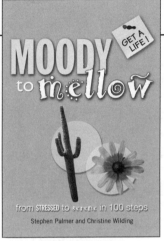

MOODY to MELLOW

0-340-90801-7

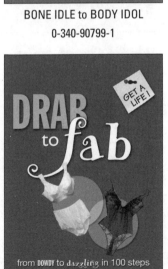

DRAB to FAB

0-340-90804-1

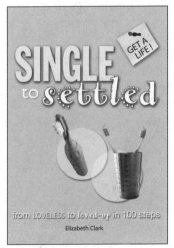

SINGLE to SETTLED

0-340-90800-9

Your notes

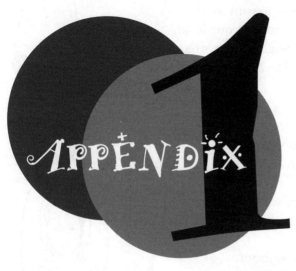

APPENDIX 1

EXERCISES

Stretching exercises

Neck stretch

1. Either standing or sitting, clasp your fingers together.
2. Drop your chin to your chest.
3. Put your hands behind your head.
4. Fully relax your head and shoulders.
5. Now apply some light pressure from your hands straight downwards to your head.
6. Breathe normally throughout the stretch.
7. Hold this stretch for 15–30 seconds.

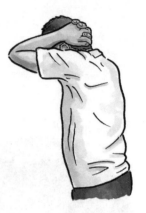

Shoulder stretch

1. Stand with your feet slightly apart, stomach tight and knees slightly bent.
2. Raise your arms above your head and put your palms together.
3. Now straighten your arms as much as is comfortable, until you feel a good stretch in your shoulders.
4. Breathe regularly throughout.
5. Hold this stretch for 15–30 seconds.

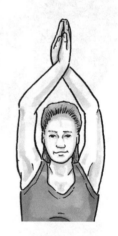

Upper arm stretch

1. Stand with your feet slightly apart, stomach tight and knees slightly bent.
2. Raise one arm and put the hand of that arm between your shoulder blades.
3. Now put your free hand on the elbow of the arm being stretched.
4. Gently ease the elbow behind your head until you feel a good stretch.
5. Breathe continuously throughout and hold for 15–30 seconds.
6. Now change sides.

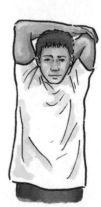

Chest stretch

1. Stand with your feet slightly apart, stomach tight and knees slightly bent.
2. Hold both hands behind your back, linking your fingers together with your palms turned in.
3. Gently raise your arms away from your body. Now bring your shoulder blades together until you feel a good stretch in your chest area.
4. Breathe regularly throughout and hold for 15–30 seconds.

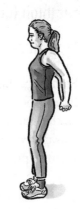

Upper back stretch

1. Stand with your feet slightly apart, stomach tight and knees slightly bent.
2. Put your arms in front of you, linking your fingers together with your palms turned in towards you.
3. Outwardly round and curve your entire back area.
4. Gently push your arms forward and away from your body until you feel a good stretch in the whole of your back area.
5. Breathe regularly throughout and hold the stretch for 15–30 seconds.

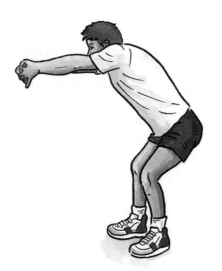

Front thigh (quad) stretch

1. For support, hold onto a steady surface.
2. Standing, slightly bend one leg.
3. Raise the other leg up and grasp the ankle, gently bringing your heel up towards your buttock.
4. Gently push your hips forward and ease the raised leg backwards until you feel a good stretch.
5. Hold this for 15–30 seconds and breathe regularly throughout.
6. Now change to the other leg.

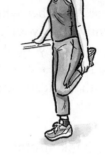

Rear thigh (hamstring) stretch

1. Put one foot forward and slightly flex the foot.
2. Bend your rear leg slightly.
3. Put your hands on your thighs and lean gently forward until you feel a good stretch along the length of the rear thigh muscles.
4. Hold this stretch for 15–30 seconds and breathe regularly throughout.
5. Now change to the other leg.

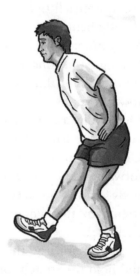

EXERCISES

Lower leg (calf) stretch

1. Find a solid, steady area to brace yourself against.
2. Put one leg forward and bend your knee slightly.
3. Keep the rear leg fairly straight.
4. Lean forward and/or move your legs further apart to increase the degree of the stretch.
5. Hold this stretch for 15–30 seconds and breathe regularly throughout.
6. Now change to the other leg.

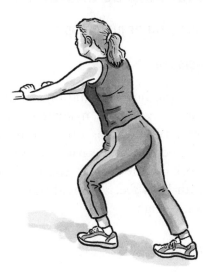

Warming up exercises

Skipping or jump-roping

Equipment

You can buy skipping ropes from any sports shop and they come in various guises – nylon/cotton, leather or a very flexible plastic material known as a speed rope. The latter two are usually better and more durable. Alternatively, use a length of cord from your garage! To work out the correct length of rope for your height, stand on the rope with both feet and hold the ends in each hand. The rope should be waist height.

Purpose

Skipping is a dynamic, entertaining and graceful form of exercise either as a warm-up or stand-alone aerobic workout. Skipping is quite demanding aerobically, so is only suitable when you've got an established exercise regime. At earlier stages, you can perform light skipping techniques with an imaginary rope!

Technique

1. Start with the rope behind you.
2. As you swing the rope in a forward motion over your head, jump slightly off the floor allowing the rope to swing freely under your feet.
3. Always rotate your wrist and not your shoulders (a common mistake) to get the flow of the swing.
4. For a warm-up, you may want to try blocks of 15–20 revolutions with a small pause in between – otherwise you'll be breathless even before you start!

EXERCISES

On-the-spot marching and jogging

You can do this exercise anywhere without any equipment!

Technique

1. To start, just march or lightly bounce from one leg to the next. One foot should always be in contact with the floor and land softly while making sure the heel of your foot presses down.
2. Swing your arms across your body, as though you're marching or jogging, as you jog on the spot.

Step-ups

Equipment

Find a suitable platform. Your knees shouldn't bend greater than a right angle as you step up.

Technique

1. Start stepping up at a slow to moderate pace, making sure you put your foot securely on the platform to help you keep your balance.
2. You can either alternate legs with each step or perform a set number of step–ups with each leg in turn.

EXERCISES

Main exercises

Don't lock!

Most toning/strength exercises involve bending and extending the joints to create the full range of movement. But try not to fully extend the joints or 'lock them out' as this places unnecessary stress on the joint and can cause injury. Your pace should be steady and smooth with no jerking or forcing. Remember, for maximum benefit, adopt the 'uncomfortably comfortable' approach.

Breathing

Breathing is one of the many naturally involuntary processes of your body. When you do toning and strengthening exercises, it's easy to overlook your breathing technique because you're concentrating on getting your posture and technique right. You only realise it when your face is turning the colour of a strawberry! When doing the exercises, try to remember to breathe out at the start of an exercise (the hardest part) and breathe in on the return (the easiest part).

The exercises described here have been split into three groups, which target different parts of the body:

◆ Upper body
◆ Mid body
◆ Lower body.

The exercises are then arranged alphabetically within each group.

Upper body exercises

Chair/bench arm dips

Purpose

This exercise targets the chest, arms and shoulders.

Technique

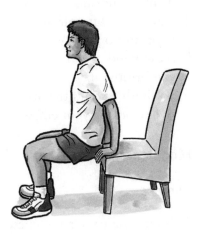

- Find a safe, solid chair, bench or edge of the bed (the height doesn't matter).
- Facing away from the support, put your hands over the edge of the seat or bench, roughly hip-width apart.
- Move slightly away from the support making sure your body weight is evenly distributed over your arms and feet.
- Keep your hips low, bend your knees and look straight ahead.
- Bend your elbows to a right angle keeping them partially tucked in as you breathe in.
- To complete the movement, semi-extend the arms as you breathe out.

Floor arm dips

Purpose

This exercise targets the back of the upper arms and shoulders.

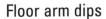

Technique

1. Sit on the floor, with your knees bent, and with feet flat and slightly apart.
2. Rest back on your hands with your palms flat.
3. Put your hands roughly hip-width apart, with your fingers turning outwards slightly.
4. Raise your hips off the floor as far as you can without arching your back, and tighten your stomach muscles.
5. Now bend at your elbows to lower your buttocks to the floor as you breathe in.
6. To finish, extend the arms as you breathe out.
7. Avoid locking your elbows and thrusting the hips during the exercise.

Modified floor press up

Purpose

This exercise targets the chest, arms and shoulders.

Technique

1. Position yourself on all fours, forming a 'box' shape with your body.
2. Put your hands slightly wider than shoulder-width apart, your knees directly under the hips and your head up slightly.
3. Now bend at the elbows to lower your chest towards the floor.
4. Keep a straight, flat back throughout the movement.
5. Your elbows should naturally move outwards.
6. Now breathe in.
7. To return, gradually extend the arms as you breathe out.

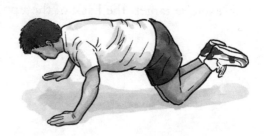

Wall press up

Purpose

This exercise targets the chest area, back of the arms and the shoulders.

Technique

1. Stand about 75cm away from a wall, facing it, with your feet slightly apart.
2. Put the palms of your hands against the wall, at shoulder height, and slightly wider than shoulder-width apart.
3. Now bend at your elbows to a right angle and breathe in.
4. To return, breathe out as you extend your arms without locking them.
5. Keep your stomach muscles tight and your back straight throughout the exercise.

Weighted arm curls

Purpose

This exercise targets the front of the arms.

Technique

1. Use a set of light weights, tin cans or bottles of water.
2. With the weights in your hands, palms facing up, stand with your feet apart and knees slightly bent.
3. Keep your back straight and stomach muscles tight.
4. Tuck your elbows into the sides of your body and extend your arms.

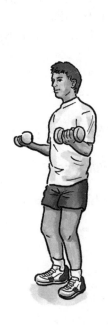

EXERCISES

265

5. Gradually curl up the weights to bend each arm fully as you breathe out.
6. Lower and extend your arms to return to the starting position as you breathe in.

Weighted arm extension

Purpose

This exercise targets the back of the upper arms.

Technique

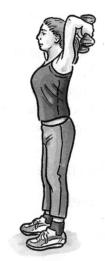

1. Use a set of light weights, tin cans or bottles of water.
2. With the weights in your hands and palms facing in towards each other, stand with your feet apart and knees slightly bent.
3. Raise the weights above your head and keep your stomach muscles tight. Remember to avoid locking your arms.
4. Bend at your elbows to lower the weight behind your head as you breathe in.
5. To complete the exercise, semi-extend your arms to the starting position above your head as you breathe out.

Weighted bent-over rows

Purpose

This exercise targets the upper back.

Technique

1. Use a set of light weights, tins cans or bottles of water.
2. Stand with your feet slightly apart and knees bent.
3. Bend your upper body forward slightly.
4. Keep a straight back and your stomach muscles tight throughout.
5. Look forward slightly and start with your arms extended in front of you and towards the floor, and palms turned in.
6. Gently pull up the weights towards your sides in the direction of your ribcage until your elbows go up past your ribs. Now breathe out.
7. Now lower the weights to the starting position as you breathe in.

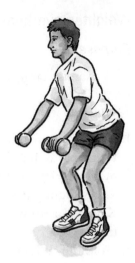

Weighted front raise

Purpose

This exercise targets the front shoulders.

Technique

1. Use a set of light weights, tin cans or bottles of water.
2. Keep your feet slightly apart and bend your knees.
3. Keep a straight back and your stomach muscles tight throughout.
4. Hold the weights in front of you, palms facing downwards, at upper thigh level.
5. Keep your elbows slightly bent.
6. Now gently raise the weights upwards to shoulder level as you breathe out.
7. Slowly lower the weights to the starting position as you breathe in.

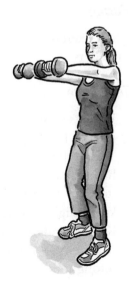

EXERCISES

Weighted overhead press

Purpose

This exercise targets the front shoulders.

Technique

1. Use a set of light weights, tin cans or bottles of water.
2. Stand upright with your feet apart and knees slightly bent.
3. Keep your stomach muscles tight all the time.
4. Hold the weights at shoulder level, with your palms facing forward and away from the body, and keep your back straight.
5. Extend your arms and weights above your head until they almost meet at the top, then breathe out.
6. Breathe in as you return the weights to shoulder level.

Weighted side raise

Purpose

This exercise targets the side shoulders.

Technique

1. Use a set of light weights, tin cans or bottles of water.
2. With the weights in your hands, palms facing inwards, stand with your feet apart and knees slightly bent.
3. Keep a straight back and your stomach muscles tight throughout.

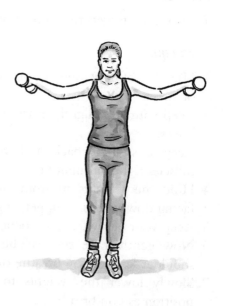

4. Hold the weights at your sides with your elbows slightly bent.
5. Now gently raise the weights sideways and upwards to shoulder level as you breathe out.
6. Slowly lower the weights to the starting position as you breathe in.

Mid body exercises

Abdominal curls

Purpose

This exercise targets the stomach.

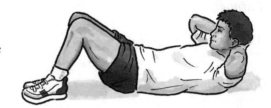

Technique

1. Lie on your back with your head back and knees bent and slightly apart.
2. Put your hands behind your ears to support your head.
3. Keep a tennis-ball-size gap between chin and chest throughout.
4. As you raise your head and shoulders until your shoulder blades are off the floor, draw in your stomach and breathe out.
5. Breathe in as you lower back to the starting position.

Abdominal reverse curls

Purpose

This exercise targets the stomach.

Technique

1. Lying on your back, lift and keep your legs straight at a right angle to your body.
2. Keep your head back, feet together and hands under your head for comfort.

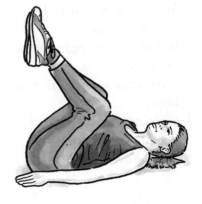

EXERCISES

269

3. Gently squeeze in your stomach muscles as you bend your knees slightly towards your chest.
4. Make sure you keep your head on the floor.
5. Your buttocks and hips should lift off the floor slightly as you breathe out.
6. Now return your legs to the starting position as you breathe in.

Bicycle abs

Purpose

This exercise targets the stomach.

Technique

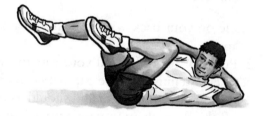

1. Lie on your back and raise both legs slightly off the floor, keeping the knees bent slightly at the start.
2. Support your head with your hands behind your ears.
3. Raise and keep your head and shoulders off the floor throughout this exercise.
4. Create a subtle twisting action with your upper body as your right elbow meets your left knee.
5. Your right leg should be semi-extended at this point, leaving the left elbow free.
6. Return your right elbow and left knee back to the starting position.
7. Now twist again so that this time your left elbow meets your right knee.
8. Continue to alternate the movements and make sure you breathe steadily throughout.
   Note: one rep = one side.

Crossover curls

Purpose

This exercise targets the stomach and waistline.

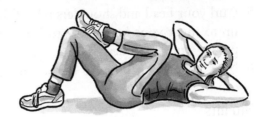

Technique

1. Lie on your back with your head back. Put your hands behind your ears – this adds good support to your head.
2. Lift one leg and place it so the ankle rests over the knee of the other leg.
3. Lift the elbow opposite the raised leg. Now curl up in a slight twisting action so that your elbow travels towards the opposite knee as you breathe out.
4. To return, lower your body to the starting position.
5. Now swap and do other side.

Curls ups

Purpose

This exercise targets the stomach.

Technique

1. Lie on your back with your head back.
2. Keeping both legs straight and together, lift them at a right angle to your body.
3. Put your hands behind your ears, adding support to your head.
4. Keep a tennis-ball-size gap between your chin and chest throughout.

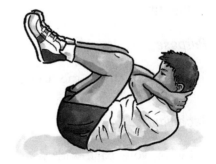

EXERCISES

5. Curl your head and shoulders up off the floor as your elbows come up to meet your knees. Try to lead with your elbows, rather than pulling your legs forward. Draw in your stomach and breathe out.
6. Now lower your body to the starting position, as you breathe in.

Hip lifts

Purpose

This exercise targets the stomach.

Technique

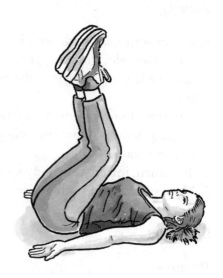

1. Lying on your back, with your head back, put your hands at your sides, with your palms facing upwards.
2. Breathe out as you draw in your stomach muscles, gently raising your legs upwards by about 5cm until your hips are slightly off the floor.
3. Keep your head back throughout and your legs straight.
4. Gently lower your hips and buttocks to the starting position as you breathe in to complete the exercise.

Pelvic tilt

Purpose

This exercise targets the stomach and lower back.

Technique

1. Lie on your back with your head back, knees bent and your arms at your sides.
2. Keep your feet slightly apart.

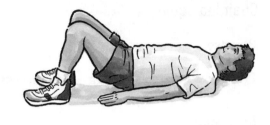

3. Now slowly rotate your hips upwards as you press your lower back into the floor. The top part of your buttocks will raise slightly off the ground.

4. Hold momentarily as you breathe out.

5. Now relax your stomach to return to the starting position and breathe in.

Lower body exercises

Alternate leg lunge

Purpose

This exercise targets the legs and buttocks.

Technique

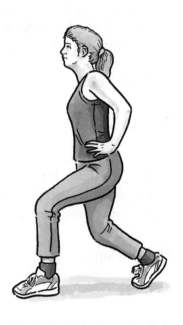

1. Stand upright with your hands on your hips or waist.

2. Step forward a minimum of 75cm with one leg, bending at the knee to no lower than a right angle.

3. The rear leg will naturally bend to the same degree and the heel of the back leg will lift off the floor.

4. Now breathe in.

5. Ensure that both feet are facing forwards.

6. Push backwards with the front leg, until you are back in the starting position and exhale here.

7. Now change to the other leg to complete the exercise.

   Note: one rep = one side.

EXERCISES

Chair leg squat

Purpose

This exercise targets the legs and buttocks.

Technique

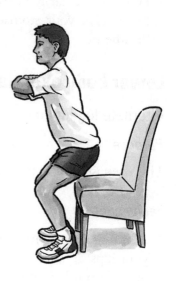

1. Find a suitable chair or other piece of furniture.
2. Stand with the chair facing forwards behind you, with your feet slightly wider than hip-width apart.
3. Turn your feet slightly outwards.
4. Cross your arms in front of your chest.
5. Now bend your knees so that your buttocks gently touch the chair.
6. As you bend, your upper body will naturally tilt forward.
7. Keep a straight back and look straight ahead throughout. Breathe in here.
8. To return, straighten your legs, making sure your knees don't lock. Now breathe out.

Full leg squat

This is the same as the half leg squat exercise below, but when you lower your buttocks, bend your knees so that your thights are almost at a right angle to the floor. Hold this position. Do not bend any further otherwise damage will occur to the knee joints!

Half leg squat

Purpose

This exercise targets the legs and buttocks.

Technique

1. Stand with your feet slightly wider than hip-width apart.
2. Turn your feet slightly outwards.
3. Cross your arms in front of your chest.
4. To lower, bend at your knees and lower your buttocks.
5. As you bend, your upper body will naturally tilt forward.
6. Keep a straight back and look straight ahead throughout the movement. Breathe in here.
7. To return, straighten your legs, making sure your knees don't lock. Now breathe out.

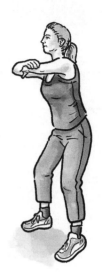

Static wall squat

Purpose

This exercise targets the upper thighs and buttocks.

Technique

1. Stand upright with your back against the wall.
2. Put your feet about hip-width apart.
3. Lower yourself by bending your knees so that your legs form a right angle to your body.
4. Make sure you breathe steadily throughout the exercise.
5. Hold this position for the required time.

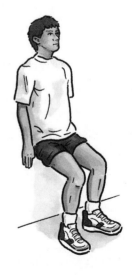

EXERCISES

Your notes

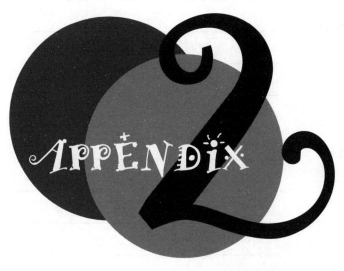

APPENDIX

DAILY RECORDS

Daily records

Food for the day

Record everything – including fluids!

Breakfast _____

_____

Mid morning snacks _____

_____

Lunch _____

_____

Afternoon snacks _____

_____

Evening meal _____

_____

Light night-time snacks _____

_____

Extras _____

_____

My fitness goal for today is: _____

_____

_____

_____

Exercise scale

Record how you felt when performing the exercises.

☐ Very tough going

☐ Fairly tough going

☐ Just about right

☐ Fairly easy

☐ Very easy

☐ Could do it with my eyes closed!

Mood of the day

Mood at start of the day

☐ Very upbeat and positive

☐ Fairly upbeat and generally happy

☐ OK

☐ A bit down

☐ Down in the dumps and depressed

Mood at the end of the day

☐ Very upbeat and positive

☐ Fairly upbeat and generally happy

☐ OK

☐ A bit down

☐ Down in the dumps and depressed

Your notes

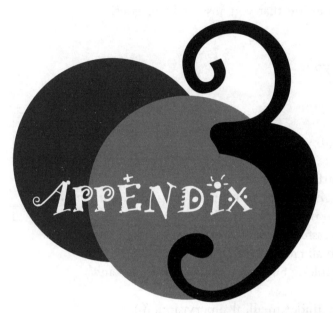

APPENDIX

QUESTIONNAIRES
AND TESTS

Pre-exercise questionnaire

Make sure that you take time to read all of the questions first. Be honest with yourself and think each one question through carefully before answering it. Circle or tick the most appropriate statement that you think best describes you. The numbers in brackets indicate your scores for every question that you answer. Here goes!

1. How old are you?
- Below 20 (3)   ☐
- 21 to 30 (2)   ☐
- 31 to 40 (1)   ☐
- 41 upwards (0)   ☐

2. Your heart and respiratory system
- I don't have any history of heart or lung disease myself or within my immediate family. (3)   ☐
- I've had successful treatment in the past and the doctor has given me the all clear. (2)   ☐
- I've got a problem, but don't receive treatment any more. (1)   ☐
- I'm currently under medical supervision. (0)   ☐

3. Your muscles and joints
- I'm currently injury free. (3)   ☐
- I've recovered from an old past injury, with no recurrence. (2)   ☐
- I'm recovering from a recent injury. (1)   ☐
- I'm currently suffering from a painful injury. (0)   ☐

4. Overall health
- My general health is good, with no signs of illness. (3)   ☐
- I'm suffering a bit with ill health, but recovering. (2)   ☐
- I'm particularly limited by illness. (1)   ☐
- I can't do much without feeling the effect of my illness. (0) ☐

5. Your weight
Weigh yourself first using accurate scales. Then using the weight chart on the next page, determine your ideal weight.

- ◆ I'm within 1 kg of my ideal weight. (3) ☐
- ◆ I'm within 4 kg of my ideal weight. (2) ☐
- ◆ I'm 5–9 kg above or below my ideal weight. (1) ☐
- ◆ I'm 10 or more kg above or below my ideal weight. (0) ☐

6. Smoking
- ◆ I don't smoke and never have. (3) ☐
- ◆ I used to smoke, but have given up. (2) ☐
- ◆ I'm a social, occasional smoker. (1) ☐
- ◆ I smoke regularly and have done for over a year. (0) ☐

7. A healthy, balanced diet?
- ◆ I eat three regular, healthy, balanced meals every day that include fresh produce, lean meat, poultry, fish, carbohydrates and water. (3) ☐
- ◆ I skip the odd meal here and there, only have a few pieces of fresh food, and don't drink lots of water. (2) ☐
- ◆ I skip breakfast and my lunch and evening meals aren't always sensible choices. (1) ☐
- ◆ I'm very erratic, mainly eating ready-made meals with no fresh produce, washed down with fizzy drinks or wine. (0) ☐

8. Exercise
- ◆ I'm currently exercising fairly briskly three or more times a week. (3) ☐
- ◆ I'm physically active on most days, for example walking the dog or doing house chores. (2) ☐
- ◆ Occasionally, I play the odd game of sport or go for a walk. (1) ☐
- ◆ I have a completely sedentary lifestyle with no exercise at all. (0) ☐

Score: _____   END OF TEST

QUESTIONNAIRES AND TESTS

Personal wellness and monitoring test

If you feel any discomfort, dizziness or nausea during the physical parts of this fitness test, then stop immediately and consult your doctor.

Ideal height to weight chart for average frame men and women

Height in cm	Weight in kg		Height in feet and inches	Weight in pounds	
	Men	Women		Men	Women
147	–	45–59	4ft 10"	–	100–131
150	–	45–60	4ft 11"	–	101–134
152	–	46–62	5ft	–	103–137
155	55–66	47–63	5ft 1"	123–145	105–140
157	56–67	49–65	5ft 2"	125–148	108–144
160	57–68	50–67	5ft 3"	127–151	111–148
162	58–70	51–69	5ft 4"	129–155	114–152
165	59–72	53–70	5ft 5"	131–159	117–156
167	60–74	54–72	5ft 6"	133–163	120–160
170	61–75	55–74	5ft 7"	135–167	123–164
172	62–77	57–75	5ft 8"	137–171	126–167
175	63–79	58–77	5ft 9"	139–175	129–170
177	64–81	60–78	5ft 10"	141–179	132–173
180	65–83	61–80	5ft 11"	144–183	135–176
182	66–85	–	6ft	147–187	–
185	68–87	–	6ft 1"	150–192	–
187	69–89	–	6ft 2"	153–197	–
190	71–91	–	6ft 3"	157–202	–

Record your weight here:

Date/weight: _____

Date/weight: _____

Date/weight: _____

Date/weight: _____

Body dimensions

Review your body dimensions on a regular basis and record them on the chart.

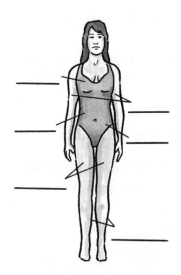

Waist-to-hip ratio

Scientists claim that there is an increased risk of suffering from certain cancers if the measurement of your waist is greater than that of your hips. If your waist is bigger than your hips, do something about it now!

Body Mass Index test (BMI)

This is a more accurate method of determining the correct weight for your height.

BMI formula:

$$\frac{\text{Weight in kilos}}{(\text{Height in m})^2}$$

For example, for a man 1.75m tall, weighing 78kg, the calculation would be:

78kg divided by 3.06m (1.75 × 1.75) = BMI of 25.49.

(To convert pounds to kilos multiply by 0.45. To convert inches to metres multiply by 0.025.)

BMI rating and scores

The recommended BMI for men is between 21–26, and for women between 18–23. Workout your own BMI rating and scores.

Women
18–23 Normal (3)   ☐
24–27 Below normal (2)   ☐
28–32 Poor (1)   ☐
33–37 Very poor (0)   ☐

Men
21–26 Normal (3)   ☐
27–30 Below normal (2)   ☐
31–34 Poor (1)   ☐
35–38 Very poor (0)   ☐

Record your BMI readings here:

Date/index: _____

Date/index: _____

Date/index: _____

Date/index: _____

Checking your level of fat

- I have a flat stomach with no love handles. (3) ☐
- I can pinch more than an inch, but less than two inches on any part of my waistline. (2) ☐
- I can grab more than a handful of soft flesh from my 'love handles'. (1) ☐
- From a standing position, I can't see my toes without bending forward. (0) ☐

Testing your cardiovascular fitness

Measuring your resting heart/pulse rate

Before you start this test, make sure that you are confident about checking your pulse rate manually. Sit down in a comfortable chair. Avoid any exciting or stressful distractions – environmental or emotional. Wait a few minutes and then check your resting heart rate. You may want to try a few times over a 10-minute period. If your readings are variable, take the average.

QUESTIONNAIRES AND TESTS

▶

287

Here's how you do it:

1. You'll need a watch or clock with a second hand or counter.
2. Using the fingers (not the thumb) of one hand, press firmly on the wrist of the other hand, about 2cm or 1 inch down from the base of the thumb. There's also a pulse along the side of your neck if you have trouble finding the pulse in your wrist.
3. Take a 15-second heartbeat count and always count your first beat as 0 then 1, 2, 3 and so on.
4. Multiply the result by 4 to find your heart rate. For example, if your 15-second heartbeat count is 20, your heart rate is 80 beats per minute (BPM).

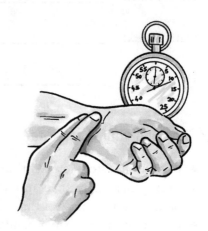

Resting heart rates and scores

60 BPM or below	Excellent (4)	☐
61–70 BPM	Good (3)	☐
71–75 BPM	Average (2)	☐
76–80 BPM	Below average (1)	☐
81–90 BPM	Poor (0)	☐

Record your resting heart rate (RHR) readings here:

Date/RHR: _____

Date/RHR: _____

Date/RHR: _____

Date/RHR: _____

The step test

This test is designed to measure your cardiovascular endurance.

- This part of the test requires light to moderate effort and some flexibility. To minimise the risk of injury you *must* make sure that you prepare your body by doing a few warm-up exercises before starting the test (see Appendix 1 on warming up and stretching).
- Before you begin the test, ensure that you are confident about checking your pulse rate manually.
- Perform the test gently without any abrupt movement.
- If you feel a burning sensation or pain in the back of your legs or elsewhere, stop. Carrying on may result in injury.

Start stepping

1. Find a suitable platform (or a similar sized stair in your home), where you can perform this test. It should be between 30cm (12 inches) and 40cm (16 inches) high.
2. Keep your back straight and stomach muscles tucked in.
3. For balance, keep your hands by your side or on your hips.
4. Step up on the platform with your entire foot. Be careful not to under or overstep the platform.
5. Start stepping up and down at a steady pace for one and a half minutes. Step up with your right foot first and then the left. Step down with your right foot followed by your left foot (right foot up, left up, right foot down and left down). Try to keep a steady, four-beat cycle. It's easy to keep up if you say, 'Up, up, down, down'.
6. Without stopping, change legs so you step up with the left foot first. Carry on for another one and a half minutes.
7. Breathe normally throughout the test.

When you've finished the test, immediately check your heart rate by taking your pulse for one minute. Compare your result to the chart on the next page.

QUESTIONNAIRES AND TESTS

▶

3-minute step test result chart (women)

Age	18–25	26–35	36–45	46–55	56–65	65+
Excellent	<85	<88	<90	<94	<95	<90
Good	85–98	88–99	90–102	94–104	95–104	90–102
Above average	99–108	100–111	103–110	105–115	105–112	103–115
Average	109–117	112–119	111–118	116–120	113–118	116–122
Below average	118–126	120–126	119–128	121–129	119–128	123–128
Poor	127–140	127–138	129–140	130–135	129–139	129–134
Very poor	>140	>138	>140	>135	>139	>134

3-minute step test result chart (men)

Age	18–25	26–35	36–45	46–55	56–65	65+
Excellent	<79	<81	<83	<87	<86	<88
Good	79–89	81–89	83–96	87–97	86–97	88–96
Above average	90–99	90–99	97–103	98–105	98–103	97–103
Average	100–105	100–107	104–112	106–116	104–112	104–113
Below average	106–116	108–117	113–119	117–122	113–120	114–120
Poor	117–128	118–128	120–130	123–132	121–129	121–130
Very poor	>128	>128	>130	>132	>129	>130

Record your heart rate (HR) readings here:

Date/HR: _____

Date/HR: _____

Date/HR: _____

Date/HR: _____

Ratings and scores

Good/excellent (3)   ☐
Average/above average (2)   ☐
Poor/below average (1)   ☐
Very poor (0)   ☐

Muscular strength and endurance test

This part of your personal fitness test aims to find out how strong you are and test your endurance by using three key exercises:

- The press up – testing your general upper condition
- The basic curl up – checking out the condition of your mid section
- The full leg squat – testing lower body strength.

You should be warmed up enough from having done the aerobic step test. But if your body's cooled down, then do some of the simple warm up exercises and stretches from Appendix 1.

Work at a pace that's both comfortable and safe – this isn't a competition! There's no time limit for finishing any of these tests. Do as many repetitions as you can and take a rest between reps if you need to. Once you've stopped each exercise, take a 30–45 second break, and then move onto the next exercise. Once you've done all three, you've finished the test. Then note down your results.

It's essential to get your posture and technique right throughout each exercise. Make sure you breathe normally. The correct breathing procedure is breathing out on exertion (for example, lifting your feet up) and breathing in on the return of every exercise (for example, putting your feet back down).

QUESTIONNAIRES AND TESTS

▶

Modified press ups. See how many you can do (see Appendix 1 for details of how to perform this exercise).

Record your results here:

Date/number: _____

Date/number: _____

Date/number: _____

Date/number: _____

Curl ups. See how many you can do (see Appendix 1 for details of how to perform this exercise).

Record your results here:

Date/number: _____

Date/number: _____

Date/number: _____

Date/number: _____

Full leg squats. See how long you can hold the squat for (see Appendix 1 for details on how to perform this exercise).

Record your results here:

Date/number: _____

Date/number: _____

Date/number: _____

Date/number: _____

Scores

Modified press up

51 or more	Excellent (3)	☐
31–50	Good (2)	☐
16–30	Average (1)	☐
15 or below	Poor (0)	☐

Curl up

51 or more	Excellent (3)	☐
31–50	Good (2)	☐
16–30	Average (1)	☐
15 or below	Poor (0)	☐

Full leg squats

61 seconds and above	Excellent (3)	☐
41–60 seconds	Good (2)	☐
31–40 seconds	Average (1)	☐
0–30 seconds	Poor (0)	☐

Score: _____

END OF TEST

How well did I do?

Now add up your total score for the Pre-exercise questionnaire and Personal wellness and monitoring test and make a note below.

Total score: _____

46 points
Well done – maximum points! Your health and fitness profile is high and you're fit and ready for exercise. Your health habits are excellent and you take good care of yourself. Keep up the excellent work and avoid known health risks and you should live a long and healthy life. Carry on and set your goals even higher.

31 or more points
Well done. Your health habits are good and you take pretty good care of yourself. Review your 'wellness and monitoring test' answers and identify where you scored lowest. A little fine-tuning could get you in even better shape.

16–30 points
You ought to take stock of your current physical condition. You're heading in the right direction, but several crucial areas need your immediate attention. Review your answers to the tests and determine your weaknesses, then work at improving your health by starting to use this book straightaway!

15 points or lower
If you scored 15 points or below, then you may be at risk by doing exercise. To improve your health, take a good hard look at your health habits and overall lifestyle, then commit to making positive changes. Check with your doctor first if you need help.

Target zone chart (Day 4)

You should now know what percentage of your Max HR is your 'target' during exercise. Now we need to find out what the target translates to in terms of heart beats. On the chart below, find your age then read across to your target percentage. This is your desired training heart rate in beats per 15 seconds.

Table of aerobic target training zones									
Age range	50%	55%	60%	65%	70%	75%	80%	85%	90%
15–20	25	28	30	33	36	38	41	43	46
21–25	25	27	30	32	35	37	39	42	44
26–30	24	27	29	31	34	36	38	41	43
31–35	23	26	28	30	33	35	37	40	42
36–40	23	25	27	30	32	34	36	39	41
41–45	22	24	27	29	31	33	35	38	40
46–50	22	24	26	28	30	32	34	37	39
51–55	21	23	25	27	29	31	33	36	38
56–60	20	22	24	26	28	30	32	34	37
61–65	19	21	23	25	27	29	31	33	35

Now you can measure your heart rate during exercise and see how you're doing (see page 288 for notes of taking your own pulse). Do you need to take things easier or pick up the pace?

Note: Each number equates to your training heart-rate objective for a 15-second period during exercise. The numbers have been found by dividing the beats-per-minute values by four – so you can quickly work out, mid-exercise, whether you're within your target zone or not.

These 15-second values are estimates and averages for a given age range. There's also a degree of error in counting for only 15 seconds instead of a full 60 seconds. But this table is still accurate enough as a quick reference guide while working out!

QUESTIONNAIRES AND TESTS

Life stress test (Day 37)

1. **Two people who know you well are talking about you. Which of the following statements would they be most likely to use? (Choose as many statements as are relevant.)**

   a. 'X is very together. Nothing much seems to bother them.' ☐

   b. 'X is great. But you have to be careful what you say to them at times.' ☐

   c. 'Something always seems to be going wrong with X's life.' ☐

   d. 'X is very moody and unpredictable.' ☐

   e. 'The less I see of X the better!' ☐

2. **Are any of the following common features of your life? (Choose as many answers as are relevant.)**
   - Feeling you can hardly ever do anything right ☐
   - Feelings of being hounded, trapped or cornered ☐
   - Indigestion ☐
   - Poor appetite ☐
   - Difficulty in getting to sleep at night ☐
   - Dizzy spells or palpitations ☐
   - Sweating without exertion or in hot weather ☐
   - Panicky feelings in crowds or in confined spaces ☐
   - Tiredness and lack of energy ☐
   - Feelings of hopelessness ('what's the use of anything?') ☐
   - Faintness or feeling nauseous without any physical cause ☐
   - Extreme irritation over small things ☐
   - Inability to unwind in the evenings ☐
   - Waking regularly at night or early in the mornings ☐
   - Difficulty in making decisions ☐
   - Inability to stop thinking about problems or the day's events ☐
   - Tearfulness ☐
   - Belief that you just can't cope ☐
   - Lack of enthusiasm even for interests you usually enjoy ☐
   - Reluctance to meet new people and try new experiences ☐
   - Inability to say no when asked to do something ☐
   - Having more responsibility than you can handle ☐

3. **Are you more or less optimistic than you used to be (or about the same)?**
   a. More ☐
   b. About the same ☐
   c. Less ☐

4. **Do you enjoy watching sports?**
   a. Yes ☐
   b. No ☐

5. **Can you get up late on weekends if you want to without feeling guilty?**
   a. Yes ☐
   b. No ☐

6. **Within reasonable professional and personal limits, can you speak your mind to your boss?**
   a. Yes ☐
   b. No ☐

7. **Can you speak your mind to your colleagues?**
   a. Yes ☐
   b. No ☐

8. **Can you speak your mind to members of your family?**
   a. Yes ☐
   b. No ☐

9. **Who usually seems to be responsible for making the important decisions in your life?**
   a. You ☐
   b. Someone else ☐

10. **If criticised by superiors at work, how would you be likely to feel?**
    a. Very upset ☐
    b. Moderately upset ☐
    c. Mildly upset ☐

▶

QUESTIONNAIRES AND TESTS

11. **Do you finish your day feeling satisfied with what you've achieved at work or in the home?**
    a. Often ☐
    b. Sometimes ☐
    c. Only occasionally ☐

12. **Do you feel most of the time that there are unsettled conflicts between you and colleagues/family members?**
    a. Yes ☐
    b. No ☐

13. **Do you feel that you've got too much work to do but not enough time?**
    a. Habitually ☐
    b. Sometimes ☐
    c. Only very occasionally ☐

14. **Do you have a clear picture of what's expected of you both personally and professionally?**
    a. Mostly ☐
    b. Sometimes ☐
    c. Hardly ever ☐

15. **Would you say that generally you have enough time to spend on yourself?**
    a. Yes ☐
    b. No ☐

16. **If you want to discuss your problems with someone, can you usually find a sympathetic ear?**
    a. Yes ☐
    b. No ☐

17. **Are you reasonably on course towards achieving your major objectives in life?**
    a. Yes ☐
    b. No ☐

18. **Are you bored at work/during the day?**
    a. Often ☐
    b. Sometimes ☐
    c. Very rarely ☐

19. **Do you look forward to going into work?**
    a. Most days ☐
    b. Some days ☐
    c. Hardly ever ☐

20. **Do you feel adequately valued for your abilities and commitment in your daily life?**
    a. Yes ☐
    b. No ☐

21. **Do you feel adequately rewarded in terms of status and promotion for your abilities and commitment at work?**
    a. Yes ☐
    b. No ☐

22. **Do you feel your superiors actively hinder you in your work? Or do they actively help you in your work?**
    a. Hinder ☐
    b. Help ☐

23. **If ten years ago, you'd been able to see yourself professionally as you are now, how would you have seen yourself?**
    a. Exceeding your expectations ☐
    b. Fulfilling your expectations ☐
    c. Falling short of your expectations ☐

24. **If you had to rate how much you like yourself on a scale from 1 (least like) to 5 (most like), what would your rating be?**
    a. 1 ☐
    b. 2 ☐
    c. 3 ☐
    d. 4 ☐
    e. 5 ☐

END OF TEST

QUESTIONNAIRES AND TESTS

Scores

For every question, score according to the following key:

1. a. 0, b. 1, c. 2, d. 3, e. 4
2. Score 1 for every 'yes' answer
3. Score 0 for a. more optimistic, 1 for b. about the same, 2 for c. less optimistic
4. Score 0 for a. 'yes', 1 for b. 'no'
5. Score 0 for a. 'yes', 1 for b. 'no'
6. Score 0 for a. 'yes', 1 for b. 'no'
7. Score 0 for a. 'yes', 1 for b. 'no'
8. Score 0 for a. 'yes', 1 for b. 'no'
9. Score 0 for a. 'yourself', 1 for b. 'someone else'
10. Score 2 for a. 'very upset', 1 for b. 'moderately upset', 0 for c. 'mildly upset'
11. Score 0 for a. 'often', 1 for b. 'sometimes', 2 for c. 'only occasionally'
12. Score 1 for a. 'yes', 0 for b. 'no'
13. Score 2 for a. 'habitually', 1 for b. 'sometimes', 0 for c. 'only very occasionally'
14. Score 0 for a. 'mostly', 1 for b. 'sometimes', 2 for c. 'hardly ever'
15. Score 0 for a. 'yes', 1 for b. 'no'
16. Score 0 for a. 'yes', 1 for b. 'no'
17. Score 0 for a. 'yes', 1 for b. 'no'
18. Score 2 for a. 'often', 1 for b. 'sometimes', 0 for c. 'very rarely'
19. Score 0 for a. 'most days', 1 for b. 'some days', 2 for c. 'hardly ever'
20. Score 0 for a. 'yes', 1 for b. 'no'
21. Score 0 for a. 'yes', 1 for b. 'no'
22. Score 1 for a. 'hinder', 0 for b. 'help'
23. Score 0 for a. 'exceeding your expectations', 1 for b. 'fulfilling your expectations', 2 for c. 'falling short of your expectations'
24. Score 4 for a. '1', 3 for b. '2', 2 for c. '3', 1 for d. '4' and 0 for e. '5'

Score: _____

Interpreting your score

Bear in mind that scores on stress scales must be interpreted cautiously. There are so many variables that lie outside the scope of these scales, but which influence the way in which we perceive and handle our stress, that two people with the same scores may think they're under quite different levels of stress. Nevertheless, if you take these scores as a guide, these scales can give us some useful information.

15 points
Stress isn't a problem in your life. But you do have enough healthy stress to keep you occupied and fulfilled.

16–30 points
This is a moderate range of stress for a busy professional. Still, it's well worth looking at how you can reasonably reduce the stress in your life.

31–45 points
Stress is clearly a problem and you need to do something about it. The longer you live with this level of stress, the harder it can become to do something about it. There's a strong case for looking carefully at your life.

45–60 points
Stress is a major problem and you must do something about it immediately. You may be nearing exhaustion. You must ease the pressure.

Your notes

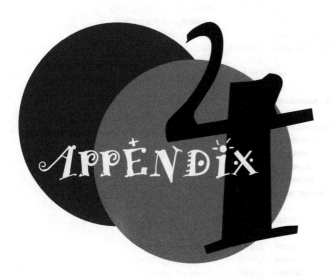

APPENDIX 4

ALL ABOUT FOOD

Food calorie chart

Note: for flour, oil and spices, calories have been given per teaspoon.

Beverages

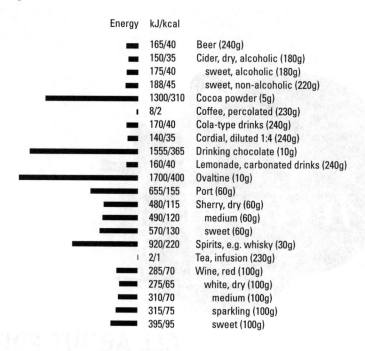

Energy	kJ/kcal	
	165/40	Beer (240g)
	150/35	Cider, dry, alcoholic (180g)
	175/40	sweet, alcoholic (180g)
	188/45	sweet, non-alcoholic (220g)
	1300/310	Cocoa powder (5g)
	8/2	Coffee, percolated (230g)
	170/40	Cola-type drinks (240g)
	140/35	Cordial, diluted 1:4 (240g)
	1555/365	Drinking chocolate (10g)
	160/40	Lemonade, carbonated drinks (240g)
	1700/400	Ovaltine (10g)
	655/155	Port (60g)
	480/115	Sherry, dry (60g)
	490/120	medium (60g)
	570/130	sweet (60g)
	920/220	Spirits, e.g. whisky (30g)
	2/1	Tea, infusion (230g)
	285/70	Wine, red (100g)
	275/65	white, dry (100g)
	310/70	medium (100g)
	315/75	sparkling (100g)
	395/95	sweet (100g)

Cereals, biscuits, cakes, deserts

Energy	kJ/kcal	
	510/120	Barley, pearl, boiled (–)
	2200/525	Biscuit, chocolate (20g)
	2095/500	cream-filled (20g)
	1365/320	crispbread, rye (20g)
	1640/390	wheat, starch-red (11g)
	1925/455	gingernut (15g)
	870/205	Bran, wheat (8g)
	1015/240	Bread, brown, slice (25g)
	1205/285	Lebanese (pita) ($\frac{1}{4}$ = 25g)
	1015/240	white, slice (25g)
	985/235	wholemeal, slice (25g)
	1230/290	roll, brown (35g)
	1630/385	starch-reduced (35g)
	1230/290	white (35g)
	1490/355	Cake, fruit (60g)
	1650/390	plain (60g)
	1940/465	sponge (60g)
	1415/335	Chapati (60g)
	1745/420	Cheesecake (120g)
	1590/380	Cornflakes (30g)
	1045/250	Crumpet (50g)
	495/120	Custard (70g)
	1200/285	Custard tart (120g)
	1465/350	Doughnut (40g)
	1570/375	Eclair (50g)
	1460/350	Flour, corn- (–)
	1505/360	plain (–)
	1525/365	self-raising (–)
	1870/445	soya, full-fat (–)
	1490/350	low-fat (–)
	1440/345	wholemeal (–)
	1555/370	Fruit pie (150g)
	1615/385	Jam tart (35g)
	250/60	Jelly, made with water (100g)
	1360/325	Lemon meringue pie (120g)
	1620/380	Meringue (15g)
	1790/425	Muesli (30g)
	625/150	Noodles (chow mein) (250g)
	1285/305	Pancake (75g)
	500/115	Pasta, macaroni, boiled (150g)
	500/115	spaghetti, boiled (120g)
	250/60	canned in tomato sauce (120g)
	2355/565	Pastry, flaky (–)
	2200/525	short crust (–)
	980/235	Pizza, cheese and tomato (150g)
	190/45	Porridge (30g)

ALL ABOUT FOOD

Cereals, biscuits, cakes, deserts continued

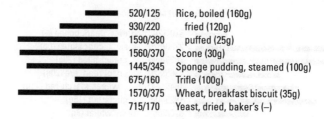

Energy kJ/kcal	
520/125	Rice, boiled (160g)
930/220	fried (120g)
1590/380	puffed (25g)
1560/370	Scone (30g)
1445/345	Sponge pudding, steamed (100g)
675/160	Trifle (100g)
1570/375	Wheat, breakfast biscuit (35g)
715/170	Yeast, dried, baker's (–)

Egg and cheese dishes

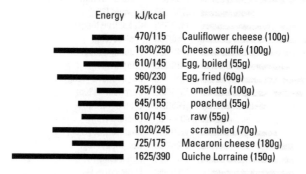

Energy	kJ/kcal	
	470/115	Cauliflower cheese (100g)
	1030/250	Cheese soufflé (100g)
	610/145	Egg, boiled (55g)
	960/230	Egg, fried (60g)
	785/190	omelette (100g)
	645/155	poached (55g)
	610/145	raw (55g)
	1020/245	scrambled (70g)
	725/175	Macaroni cheese (180g)
	1625/390	Quiche Lorraine (150g)

Fats and oils

Energy	kJ/kcal	
	3045/730	Butter, salted (10g)
	3665/990	Dripping, beef (–)
	3665/890	Lard (–)
	3045/730	Margarine (10g)
	3695/900	Vegetable oils (–)

ALL ABOUT FOOD

Fish and other seafoods

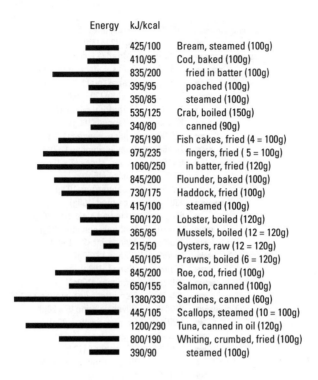

Energy	kJ/kcal	
	425/100	Bream, steamed (100g)
	410/95	Cod, baked (100g)
	835/200	fried in batter (100g)
	395/95	poached (100g)
	350/85	steamed (100g)
	535/125	Crab, boiled (150g)
	340/80	canned (90g)
	785/190	Fish cakes, fried (4 = 100g)
	975/235	fingers, fried (5 = 100g)
	1060/250	in batter, fried (120g)
	845/200	Flounder, baked (100g)
	730/175	Haddock, fried (100g)
	415/100	steamed (100g)
	500/120	Lobster, boiled (120g)
	365/85	Mussels, boiled (12 = 120g)
	215/50	Oysters, raw (12 = 120g)
	450/105	Prawns, boiled (6 = 120g)
	845/200	Roe, cod, fried (100g)
	650/155	Salmon, canned (100g)
	1380/330	Sardines, canned (60g)
	445/105	Scallops, steamed (10 = 100g)
	1200/290	Tuna, canned in oil (120g)
	800/190	Whiting, crumbed, fried (100g)
	390/90	steamed (100g)

Fruit

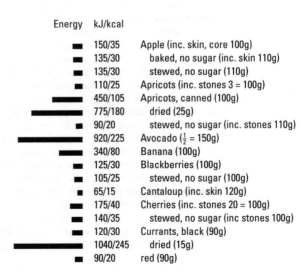

Energy	kJ/kcal	
	150/35	Apple (inc. skin, core 100g)
	135/30	baked, no sugar (inc. skin 110g)
	135/30	stewed, no sugar (110g)
	110/25	Apricots (inc. stones 3 = 100g)
	450/105	Apricots, canned (100g)
	775/180	dried (25g)
	90/20	stewed, no sugar (inc. stones 110g)
	920/225	Avocado ($\frac{1}{2}$ = 150g)
	340/80	Banana (100g)
	125/30	Blackberries (100g)
	105/25	stewed, no sugar (100g)
	65/15	Cantaloup (inc. skin 120g)
	175/40	Cherries (inc. stones 20 = 100g)
	140/35	stewed, no sugar (inc stones 100g)
	120/30	Currants, black (90g)
	1040/245	dried (15g)
	90/20	red (90g)

Fruit continued

1055/250	Dates, dried (6 = 35g)
175/40	Figs (2 = 75g)
910/215	dried (2 = 40g)
405/95	Fruit salad, canned (120g)
215/50	Grapes, black (20 = 100g)
255/60	white (20 = 100g)
45/10	Grapefruit, whole (200g)
255/60	canned (100g)
130/30	juice, canned (120g)
260/60	Guavas, canned (100g)
65/15	Lemon, slices (2 = 15g)
30/7	juice (15g)
75/15	Loganberries (100g)
430/100	canned (100g)
65/15	stewed, no sugar (100g)
290/70	Lychees, canned (100g)
195/46	Mandarins (2 = 100g)
235/55	canned (50g)
255/60	Mango (100g)
330/75	canned (100g)
200/45	Nectarines (inc. stones 3 = 100g)
340/80	Olives, in brine (5 = 20g)
115/25	Orange, whole (130g)
160/40	juice, fresh (120g)
145/35	canned (120g)
60/15	Passionfruit, whole (30g)
170/40	Papaw (100g)
275/65	canned (100g)
135/30	Peach (inc. stones 120g)
375/85	canned (120g)
905/210	dried (25g)
335/80	Peach, stewed, no sugar (120g)
125/30	Pear (inc. skin, core 120g)
325/75	canned (120g)
130/30	stewed, no sugar (120g)
195/45	Pineapple (80g)
330/75	canned (80g)
225/55	juice, canned (120g)
145/35	Plums (inc. stones 3 = 100g)
125/30	stewed, no sugar (inc. stones 100g)
570/135	Prunes (inc. stones 8 = 80g)
315/75	stewed, no sugar (inc. stones 120g)
105/25	Quince, raw (100g)
1050/245	Raisins, dried (20g)
105/25	Raspberries (100g)
370/85	canned (100g)
110/25	stewed, no sugar (100g)
25/6	Rhubarb, stewed, no sugar (120g)

Fruit continued

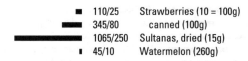

■	110/25	Strawberries (10 = 100g)
■■	345/80	canned (100g)
■■■■■■	1065/250	Sultanas, dried (15g)
▪	45/10	Watermelon (260g)

Meat and meat products

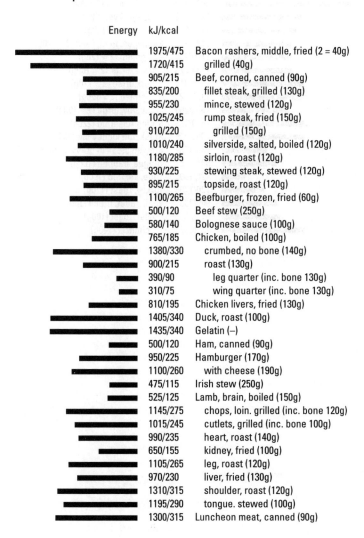

Energy	kJ/kcal	
	1975/475	Bacon rashers, middle, fried (2 = 40g)
	1720/415	grilled (40g)
	905/215	Beef, corned, canned (90g)
	835/200	fillet steak, grilled (130g)
	955/230	mince, stewed (120g)
	1025/245	rump steak, fried (150g)
	910/220	grilled (150g)
	1010/240	silverside, salted, boiled (120g)
	1180/285	sirloin, roast (120g)
	930/225	stewing steak, stewed (120g)
	895/215	topside, roast (120g)
	1100/265	Beefburger, frozen, fried (60g)
	500/120	Beef stew (250g)
	580/140	Bolognese sauce (100g)
	765/185	Chicken, boiled (100g)
	1380/330	crumbed, no bone (140g)
	900/215	roast (130g)
	390/90	leg quarter (inc. bone 130g)
	310/75	wing quarter (inc. bone 130g)
	810/195	Chicken livers, fried (130g)
	1405/340	Duck, roast (100g)
	1435/340	Gelatin (–)
	500/120	Ham, canned (90g)
	950/225	Hamburger (170g)
	1100/260	with cheese (190g)
	475/115	Irish stew (250g)
	525/125	Lamb, brain, boiled (150g)
	1145/275	chops, loin. grilled (inc. bone 120g)
	1015/245	cutlets, grilled (inc. bone 100g)
	990/235	heart, roast (140g)
	650/155	kidney, fried (100g)
	1105/265	leg, roast (120g)
	970/230	liver, fried (130g)
	1310/315	shoulder, roast (120g)
	1195/290	tongue. stewed (100g)
	1300/315	Luncheon meat, canned (90g)

ALL ABOUT FOOD

Meat and meat products continued

960/230	Meat pie (180g)
810/195	Moussaka (200g)
1390/330	Pastie (160g)
1075/260	Pork, chop, loin, grilled (100g)
1190/285	leg, roast (120g)
770/185	sweet and sour (250g)
1565/375	Pork pie (180g)
380/90	Rabbit, stewed (inc. bone 170g)
2030/490	Salami, slices (3 = 90g)
1285/310	Sausage, liver (60g)
1210/290	Sausage roll (100g)
1125/270	Sausages, beef, fried (2 = 120g)
1105/265	grilled (2 = 120g)
1135/275	frankfurter (2 = 100g)
1315/315	pork, fried (2 = 120g)
1320/320	grilled (2 = 120g)
1090/260	saveloy, large (2 = 150g)
1400/335	Spring roll, fried (220g)
1350/325	Steak and kidney pie (180g)
730/175	Stewed steak in gravy, canned (100g)
885/215	Tongue, canned (100g)
420/100	Tripe, stewed (100g)
720/170	Turkey, roast (120g)
905/230	Veal, cutlet, fried (110g)
965/230	fillet, roast (100g)
1335/320	schnitzel (140g)

Milk and milk products

Energy	kJ/kcal	
	1245/300	Cheese, camembert (25g)
	1680/405	cheddar (25g)
	1175/285	cheese spread (10g)
	400/95	cottage (25g)
	1805/440	cream cheese (15g)
	1470/355	Danish blue (25g)
	1260/305	edam (25g)
	1695/410	parmesan (10g)
	1290/310	processed (25g)
	1915/460	stilton (25g)
	1585/375	Swiss (25g)
	1525/365	Cream, 35% fat (30g)
	950/230	sterilised, canned (15g)
	705/170	Ice-cream (60g)
	690/165	non-dairy (60g)
	1140/265	Milk, cow's, cond. skim, sweet (30g)
	1360/320	cond, whole, sweet (30g)
	1510/355	dried, skimmed (12g)
	2050/490	dried, whole (10g)
	660/160	evap. whole, unsweet (30g)
	360/85	flavoured (230g)
	140/35	fresh, skimmed (230g)
	275/65	fresh, whole (230g)
	275/65	longlife, UHT (230g)
	290/70	goat's (230g)
	510/120	Milkshake, flavoured (340g)
	420/100	Yoghurt, flavoured (200g)
	405/95	fruit, low-fat (200g)
	215/50	natural, low-fat (200g)
	325/75	plain (200g)

ALL ABOUT FOOD

Nuts

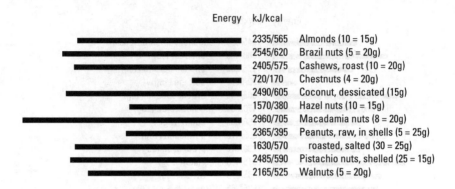

Energy	kJ/kcal	
	2335/565	Almonds (10 = 15g)
	2545/620	Brazil nuts (5 = 20g)
	2405/575	Cashews, roast (10 = 20g)
	720/170	Chestnuts (4 = 20g)
	2490/605	Coconut, dessicated (15g)
	1570/380	Hazel nuts (10 = 15g)
	2960/705	Macadamia nuts (8 = 20g)
	2365/395	Peanuts, raw, in shells (5 = 25g)
	1630/570	roasted, salted (30 = 25g)
	2485/590	Pistachio nuts, shelled (25 = 15g)
	2165/525	Walnuts (5 = 20g)

Sauces and condiments

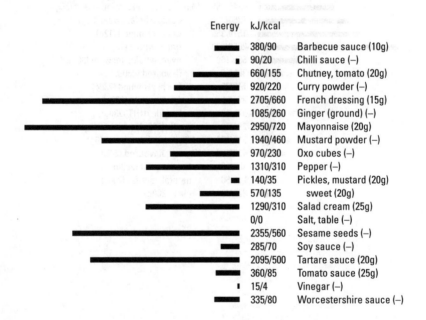

Energy	kJ/kcal	
	380/90	Barbecue sauce (10g)
	90/20	Chilli sauce (–)
	660/155	Chutney, tomato (20g)
	920/220	Curry powder (–)
	2705/660	French dressing (15g)
	1085/260	Ginger (ground) (–)
	2950/720	Mayonnaise (20g)
	1940/460	Mustard powder (–)
	970/230	Oxo cubes (–)
	1310/310	Pepper (–)
	140/35	Pickles, mustard (20g)
	570/135	sweet (20g)
	1290/310	Salad cream (25g)
	0/0	Salt, table (–)
	2355/560	Sesame seeds (–)
	285/70	Soy sauce (–)
	2095/500	Tartare sauce (20g)
	360/85	Tomato sauce (25g)
	15/4	Vinegar (–)
	335/80	Worcestershire sauce (–)

ALL ABOUT FOOD

Soups

Energy	kJ/kcal	
	205/50	Chicken, condensed (230g)
	85/20	Chicken noodle, dried (230g)
	100/25	Minestrone, dried (230g)
	220/55	Mushroom, canned (230g)
	260/60	Tomato, condensed (230g)
	130/30	Tomato, dried (230g)
	160/35	Vegetable, canned (230g)

Sugars, jams and spreads

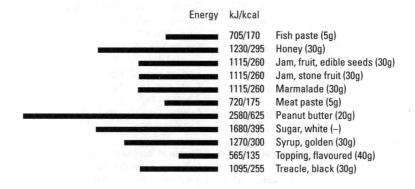

Energy	kJ/kcal	
	705/170	Fish paste (5g)
	1230/295	Honey (30g)
	1115/260	Jam, fruit, edible seeds (30g)
	1115/260	Jam, stone fruit (30g)
	1115/260	Marmalade (30g)
	720/175	Meat paste (5g)
	2580/625	Peanut butter (20g)
	1680/395	Sugar, white (–)
	1270/300	Syrup, golden (30g)
	565/135	Topping, flavoured (40g)
	1095/255	Treacle, black (30g)

Sweets

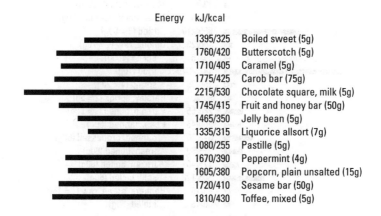

Energy	kJ/kcal	
	1395/325	Boiled sweet (5g)
	1760/420	Butterscotch (5g)
	1710/405	Caramel (5g)
	1775/425	Carob bar (75g)
	2215/530	Chocolate square, milk (5g)
	1745/415	Fruit and honey bar (50g)
	1465/350	Jelly bean (5g)
	1335/315	Liquorice allsort (7g)
	1080/255	Pastille (5g)
	1670/390	Peppermint (4g)
	1605/380	Popcorn, plain unsalted (15g)
	1720/410	Sesame bar (50g)
	1810/430	Toffee, mixed (5g)

ALL ABOUT FOOD

Vegetables

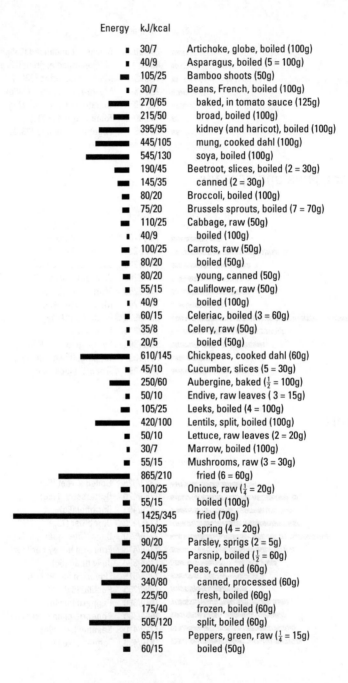

Energy	kJ/kcal	
	30/7	Artichoke, globe, boiled (100g)
	40/9	Asparagus, boiled (5 = 100g)
	105/25	Bamboo shoots (50g)
	30/7	Beans, French, boiled (100g)
	270/65	baked, in tomato sauce (125g)
	215/50	broad, boiled (100g)
	395/95	kidney (and haricot), boiled (100g)
	445/105	mung, cooked dahl (100g)
	545/130	soya, boiled (100g)
	190/45	Beetroot, slices, boiled (2 = 30g)
	145/35	canned (2 = 30g)
	80/20	Broccoli, boiled (100g)
	75/20	Brussels sprouts, boiled (7 = 70g)
	110/25	Cabbage, raw (50g)
	40/9	boiled (100g)
	100/25	Carrots, raw (50g)
	80/20	boiled (50g)
	80/20	young, canned (50g)
	55/15	Cauliflower, raw (50g)
	40/9	boiled (100g)
	60/15	Celeriac, boiled (3 = 60g)
	35/8	Celery, raw (50g)
	20/5	boiled (50g)
	610/145	Chickpeas, cooked dahl (60g)
	45/10	Cucumber, slices (5 = 30g)
	250/60	Aubergine, baked ($\frac{1}{2}$ = 100g)
	50/10	Endive, raw leaves (3 = 15g)
	105/25	Leeks, boiled (4 = 100g)
	420/100	Lentils, split, boiled (100g)
	50/10	Lettuce, raw leaves (2 = 20g)
	30/7	Marrow, boiled (100g)
	55/15	Mushrooms, raw (3 = 30g)
	865/210	fried (6 = 60g)
	100/25	Onions, raw ($\frac{1}{4}$ = 20g)
	55/15	boiled (100g)
	1425/345	fried (70g)
	150/35	spring (4 = 20g)
	90/20	Parsley, sprigs (2 = 5g)
	240/55	Parsnip, boiled ($\frac{1}{2}$ = 60g)
	200/45	Peas, canned (60g)
	340/80	canned, processed (60g)
	225/50	fresh, boiled (60g)
	175/40	frozen, boiled (60g)
	505/120	split, boiled (60g)
	65/15	Peppers, green, raw ($\frac{1}{4}$ = 15g)
	60/15	boiled (50g)

Vegetables continued

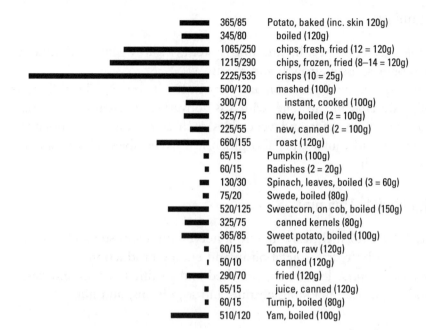

	365/85	Potato, baked (inc. skin 120g)
	345/80	boiled (120g)
	1065/250	chips, fresh, fried (12 = 120g)
	1215/290	chips, frozen, fried (8–14 = 120g)
	2225/535	crisps (10 = 25g)
	500/120	mashed (100g)
	300/70	instant, cooked (100g)
	325/75	new, boiled (2 = 100g)
	225/55	new, canned (2 = 100g)
	660/155	roast (120g)
	65/15	Pumpkin (100g)
	60/15	Radishes (2 = 20g)
	130/30	Spinach, leaves, boiled (3 = 60g)
	75/20	Swede, boiled (80g)
	520/125	Sweetcorn, on cob, boiled (150g)
	325/75	canned kernels (80g)
	365/85	Sweet potato, boiled (100g)
	60/15	Tomato, raw (120g)
	50/10	canned (120g)
	290/70	fried (120g)
	65/15	juice, canned (120g)
	60/15	Turnip, boiled (80g)
	510/120	Yam, boiled (100g)

ALL ABOUT FOOD

Vitamins and their food sources

Vitamin A

Needed for: eye health, immune system, healthy skin and mucous membranes, tissue growth and repair

Best food sources: Foods contain very little vitamin A. The following foods are rich in carotene, which is converted to vitamin A: orange, red and yellow fruit and vegetables such as carrots, sweet potatoes, tomatoes and cantaloupe; also green leafy vegetables such as spinach and broccoli

Vitamin B1 (Thiamin)

Needed for: normal heart function, nerves, muscle tissue and digestive system, carbohydrate metabolism and energy production

Best food sources: lean meat, enriched and fortified cereals and baked foods, legumes (including peanuts and soya beans) and nuts

Vitamin B2 (Riboflavin)

Needed for: energy production, immune system, healthy skin

Best food sources: low-fat dairy products, lean meat, eggs, enriched and fortified cereals, green leafy vegetables

Vitamin B3 (Niacin)

Needed for: energy production, healthy skin and digestive system

Best food sources: The following foods are rich in the amino acid tryptophan which the body converts into niacin: lean meat, pork, veal, tuna, halibut, poultry, nuts, enriched and fortified cereals, yeast, baked potatoes, coffee and tea

Vitamin B6 (Pyrodoxine)

Needed for: energy production, red blood cell formation, immunity, nervous system and hormone function

Best food sources: lean beef, tuna, halibut, legumes, enriched and fortified cereals, leafy green vegetables

Vitamin B12

Needed for: energy production, red blood cell production, utilisation of folic acid, nervous system function
Best food sources: lean meat, poultry, fish, eggs, low-fat dairy products

Folic acid

Needed for: energy production, red blood cell formation and growth, essential for prevention of certain birth defects
Best food sources: lean meat, fish, nuts, leafy green vegetables, whole grains

Pantothenic acid

Needed for: carbohydrate, fat, energy and protein metabolism
Best food sources: widespread in the food supply, found in lean meat, fish, poultry, wholegrain cereals

Biotin

Needed for: energy production, fatty acid synthesis and the breakdown of certain amino acids
Best food sources: widespread in the food supply, but especially concentrated in egg yolks, liver, mushrooms, peanuts, yeast, milk, meat and most vegetables

Vitamin C (Ascorbic acid)

Needed for: normal growth, wound healing, disease and infection resistance, bone and teeth formation, more efficient iron absorption
Best food sources: citrus fruit, berries, potatoes, tomatoes, peppers, leafy green vegetables

ALL ABOUT FOOD

Vitamin D

Needed for: normal growth, healthy bones, teeth and nails, proper absorption of calcium and phosphorus
Best food sources: fortified milk and milk products, also synthesised in the skin when exposed to sunlight

Vitamin E (tocopherol)

Needed for: cell membrane integrity and protection
Best food sources: vegetable oils, margarine, eggs, fish, wholegrain cereals, dried beans

Vitamin K

Needed for: production of proteins required for normal blood clotting
Best food sources: leafy green vegetables and cereals, also synthesised in the digestive tract

Minerals and their food sources

Calcium

Needed for: healthy bones, teeth, nails, muscle tissue; helps in blood clotting and heart and nerve functions; recommended daily intake is higher for children, adolescents, pregnant and lactating women, and women starting menopause
Best food sources: low-fat dairy products such as skimmed milk and yoghurt; also eggs, green leafy vegetables, broccoli, canned salmon or sardines with bones

Chromium

Needed for: normal release of energy from glucose
Best food sources: nuts, cheeses and unrefined grains

Copper

Needed for: enzyme reactions, iron metabolism
Best food sources: seafood, legumes (dried beans and peas), grains, nuts, seeds and hard water

Fluoride

Needed for: healthy bones and teeth to resist decay
Best food sources: fluoridated water and toothpaste, seafood and tea; cooking foods in Teflon (a fluoride containing polymer) increases fluoride content

Iodine

Needed for: regulation of body temperature, thyroid hormone synthesis, metabolic rate, reproduction, growth and nerve and muscle function
Best food sources: seafood, iodised salt

Iron

Needed for: formation of healthy red blood cells and prevention of anaemia (helps carry oxygen to cells); recommended daily iron intake is higher for women aged 11–50 to compensate for iron loss during menstruation
Best food sources: lean red meats, shellfish, dried fruit, green leafy vegetables (iron from non-meat sources is best absorbed when vitamin C is also present)

Magnesium

Needed for: energy production, normal heart and nerve function, prevention of muscle cramps
Best food sources: green leafy vegetables, shellfish, tofu, nuts, and seeds

ALL ABOUT FOOD

Phosphorus

Needed for: growth, bone density, energy production, regulates blood chemistry
Best food sources: lean meat, fish, poultry, low-fat dairy products

Potassium

Needed for: regulation and balance of body fluids, promotes normal heart rhythm, prevents muscle cramping
Best food sources: bananas, other fruit, dried fruit, vegetables, skimmed milk

Selenium

Needed for: antioxidant properties protect vitamin E and poly-unsaturated fats in the body
Best food sources: seafood, meats, grains

Sodium

Needed for: regulation of body fluids and maintenance of acid-base balance; helps nerve transmission and muscle contraction
Best food sources: found in all foods and especially high in processed foods

Zinc

Needed for: normal appetite and taste, wound healing, healthy skin and normal growth
Best food sources: lean meat, shellfish, wheat germ, yoghurt, legumes

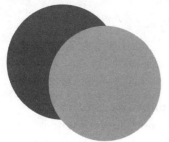

USEFUL CONTACTS

Fitness Associations

The Keep Fit Association can direct and advise on a whole range of fitness matters.
www.keepfit.org.uk

The National Register of Personal Trainers can help you to locate qualified trainers in your region, price range and needs.
www.nrpt.co.uk

Walking clubs

www.walking.timeoutdoors.com

Fitness equipment suppliers

www.fitnessnetwork.co.uk
www.fitness-superstore.co.uk

Alcoholics Anonymous

Their primary purpose is to stay sober and help other alcoholics to achieve sobriety.
www.aa-uk.org.uk
Tel: 0845 7697555

British Nutrition Foundation

Promotes the nutritional well-being of the public. It is a charitable organisation working with the food industry and government.
www.nutrition.org.uk

General Osteopathic Council

A register that lists qualified, approved osteopaths.
www.osteopathy.org.uk

The General Chiropractic Council

Keeps a register of chiropractors who meet their standards and training.
www.gcc-uk.org

Further reading

C. Chin, *Exercise for Everyone: Cornel Chin's Triple A Fitness Programme for Anyone, Anywhere, Anytime* (London, Quadrille Publishing, 2004)

K. Switzer, *Running and Walking for Women Over 40: The Road to Sanity and Vanity* (Hampshire, St. Martin's Press, 1998)

S. Whalley and L. Jackson, *Running Made Easy* (London, Robson Books Ltd, 2004)

J. Sherman-Wolin, *Smart Girls Do Dumbells* (USA, Riverhead Books U.S., 2004)

Recommended fitness magazines

Zest
Personal Trainer for Women
TopSanté